Poc

Varney's
Pocket Midwife

Helen Varney, CNM, MSN, DHL (Hon.), FACNM
Professor
Nurse-Midwifery Program
Yale University School of Nursing

Jan M. Kriebs, CNM, MSN, FACNM
Clinical Instructor
Department of Obstetrics,
Gynecology and Reproductive Sciences
University of Maryland School of Medicine

Carolyn L. Gegor, CNM, MS, RDMS
Assistant Professor
Department of Obstetrics, Gynecology and Reproductive Sciences
University of Maryland School of Medicine

JONES AND BARTLETT PUBLISHERS
Sudbury, Massachusetts
BOSTON   TORONTO   LONDON   SINGAPORE

World Headquarters
Jones and Bartlett Publishers
40 Tall Pine Drive
Sudbury, MA 01776
978-443-5000
800-832-0034
info@jbpub.com
www.jbpub.com

Jones and Bartlett Publishers Canada
P.O. Box 19020
Toronto, ON M5S 1X1
CANADA

Jones and Bartlett Publishers International
Barb House, Barb Mews
London W6 7PA
UK

Production Credits
Acquisitions Editor   Karen McClure
Production Editor   Lianne B. Ames
Manufacturing Buyer   Jane Bromback
Design   Clarinda Publication Services
Editorial Production Service   Clarinda Publication Services
Typesetting   The Clarinda Company
Cover Design   Dick Hannus
Printing and Binding   United Graphics
Cover Printing   United Graphics

Library of Congress Cataloging-in-Publication Data
Varney, Helen.
    Varney's pocket midwife / Helen Varney, Jan M. Kriebs, Carolyn L.
Gegor.
        p.   cm.
    Companion v. to: Varney's midwifery / Helen Varney. 3rd ed. c1997.
    Includes index.
    ISBN 0-7637-0546-2 (spiral bound)
    1. Midwifery.   2. Gynecologic nursing.   3. Maternity nursing.
4. Midwifery—Handbooks, manuals, etc.   5. Gynecologic nursing—
Handbooks, manuals, etc.   6. Maternity nursing—Handbooks, manuals,
etc.   I. Kriebs, Jan M.   II. Gegor, Carolyn L.   III. Varney, Helen.
Varney's midwifery.   IV. Title.
    [DNLM: 1. Midwifery—handbooks.   2. Obstetrical Nursing—
handbooks.   WY 49 V318v 1998]
RG950.V37 1997 Suppl.
618.2—dc21
DNLM/DLC
for Library of Congress   97-42676
                                                                              CIP

Contents

Introduction		vi
Chapter 1	Processes of Care	1
Chapter 2	Anatomy and Physiology	4
Chapter 3	Health Care of Well Women	13
Chapter 4	Common Health Problems	53
Chapter 5	Preconception Care	86
Chapter 6	Antepartum	89
Chapter 7	Fetal Assessment	107
Chapter 8	Nutrition in Pregnancy	125
Chapter 9	Exercise During Pregnancy	142
Chapter 10	Antepartal Complications	149
Chapter 11	Intrapartum	205
Chapter 12	Intrapartal Complications	235
Chapter 13	Postpartum	300
Chapter 14	Newborn	309
References		331
Appendix A	Sample Format for Chart Notes and Prescriptions	336
Appendix B	ACNM Documents	342
Appendix C	Street and E-mail Addresses, Telephone, FAX, and Beeper Numbers	352
Appendix D	Computer Prompts and Passwords	354
Appendix E	Certificate and License Numbers	355
Appendix F	Abbreviations and Acronyms	356
Appendix G	FDA Pregnancy Risk Categories for Drugs	363
Appendix H	Temperature Conversion Chart	364
Index		366

Introduction

Virtually every midwife we know has, at some time, carried a pocket clinical notebook. Usually begun in school, it becomes over the years a collection of those things we need to know quickly or in the middle of the night, a teaching tool for our students, an *aide memoire* when new paperwork leaves us momentarily distracted, and a reminder of rarely used facts. The contents change with time, clinical site, and skill. Sometimes, it isn't the contents but the comfort that keeps us carrying them.

With the third edition of *Varney's Midwifery,* the time seemed right for a pocket clinical notebook intended both for students and practicing midwives. *Varney's Pocket Midwife* uses *Varney's Midwifery, 3rd edition,* as the "mother book," with chapter end notes stating the page numbers from whence came the vast majority of the contents of the pocket notebook. This enables the reader to readily refer to the more comprehensive textbook for complete information Since we know that each of us keeps different items in our pocket notebook, we tried to make the contents as generally useful as possible. We have interspersed blank note pages throughout the book for your individual additions.

One word of caution is necessary. Every clinical site has its own laboratory norms, its own formulary or preferred medications, and its own arrangement for consultation. Further, recommended medications and other therapies change over time. Therefore, it is essential that each clinician check for local laboratory norms and up-to-date therapeutic recommendations.

This pocket clinical notebook was written for you. We invite your comments and suggestions of additional content, graphs, charts, and tables you think would be helpful to include, as well as what you think we could eliminate in the next edition.

Acknowledgments

We gratefully acknowledge Mary Curran LNM, MPH, for her contributions and for her support and sense of humor during the gestation of this manuscript.

We especially acknowledge the contributing authors to *Varney's Midwifery,* 3rd whose material we used in this pocket clinical notebook, as attributed in the chapter end notes.

We give special thanks to Clayton Jones, Lianne Ames, and Karen McClure of Jones and Bartlett, and to Emily Autumn of Clarinda Publication Services. Each was helpful in unique and individual ways in keeping with the much appreciated Jones and Bartlett philosophy of communicating with and involvement of authors.

HVB
JK
CG

Chapter 1

Processes of Care[1]

Management Framework: Process

1. Investigate by obtaining all necessary data for complete evaluation of the patient.
2. Make an accurate identification of problems or diagnoses based on correct interpretation of the data.
3. Anticipate other potential problems or diagnoses that might be expected because of the identified problems or diagnoses.
4. Evaluate the need for immediate midwife or physician intervention and/or for consultation or collaborative management with other health care team members, as dictated by the patient's condition.
5. Develop a comprehensive plan of care that is supported by explanations of valid rationale underlying the decisions made and is based on the preceding steps.
6. Direct or implement the plan of care efficiently and safely.
7. Evaluate the effectiveness of the care given, recycling appropriately through the management process for any aspect of care that has been ineffective.

Management Framework: Principles*

1. Minimize physical and emotional discomfort.
2. Maintain privacy to extent possible.
3. Adapt approach to consumer as appropriate.
4. Provide opportunity for consumer to receive support from significant other.
5. Exchange information in manner that consumer understands.
6. Demonstrate sensitivity to the biases and constraints of the consumer, setting, system, and health care provider.
7. Provide opportunity for asking questions.
8. Promote consumer's right to make and be responsible for decisions concerning personal health care.
9. Demonstrate awareness of cost/benefit ratio in health care.
10. Communicate appropriately with health team members, faculty, and peers.
11. Develop environment of mutual respect in any professional interaction.
12. Accept responsibility for decision-making and its consequences.
13. Identify bioethical considerations related to reproductive health.

*Source: By permission of Yale University School of Nursing, Nurse-Midwifery Program, 1997.

Management Framework: Skills*

Perform all skills in a manner that: 1. Demonstrates correct and efficient use of hands, instruments, and equipment 2. Results in obtaining accurate data 3. Results in the safe completion of an appropriate procedure or maneuver, using standard (universal) precautions 4. Causes the least possible physical and/or psychological discomfort.

Perform and explain a complete or interval physical examination, as appropriate.

Source: By permission of Yale University School of Nursing, Nurse-Midwifery Program, 1997.

The Process of Differential Diagnosis

1. Recognize a sign or symptom as either indicative of abnormality or needing further evaluation.
2. List all the possible conditions, diseases, or complications of which the sign or symptom could be indicative.
3. Go through the list methodically, obtaining additional pertinent data (from history, physical and pelvic examinations, laboratory test results, or adjunctive studies) that either confirm or rule out each condition, disease, or complication on the list.

Chapter 2

Anatomy and Physiology

◼ **Menstrual Cycle**

FSH and LH Laboratory Values*

Follicle Stimulating Hormone (FSH)

Prepubertal	<10 mlU/ml
Follicular	5–20 mlU/ml
Midcycle	15–30 mlU/ml
Luteal	5–15 mlU/ml
Menopausal	40–100 mlU/ml

Luteinizing Hormone (LH)

Follicular	2–15 mlU/ml
Ovulatory	13–145 mlU/ml
Luteal	2–15 mlU/ml
Postmenopausal	13–145 mlU/ml

Source: Used with permission from G. D. Willett. *Laboratory Testing in OB/GYN.* Boston: Blackwell Scientific Publications, 1994.

FIGURE 2-1   *Menstrual Cycle* (see p. 5)
Events of pituitary, ovarian, and menstrual cycle. Note plasma estradiol peaks about day 12, plasma follicle-stimulating hormone (FSH) and luteinizing hormone (LH) about day 13, and ovulation about day 14.

Source: Reproduced with permission from J. R. Scott, P. J. DiSaia, C. B. Hammond, and W. Spellacy, (eds). *Danforth's Obstetrics and Gynecology,* 6th ed. Philadelphia: J.B. Lippincott Company, 1990, p. 58.

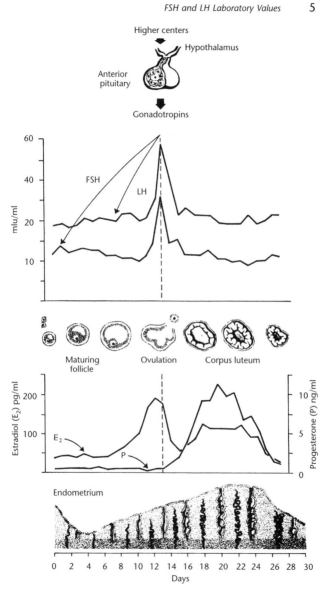

Higher centers

Hypothalamus

Anterior pituitary

Gonadotropins

Maturing follicle

Ovulation

Corpus luteum

Endometrium

Pelvic Anatomy

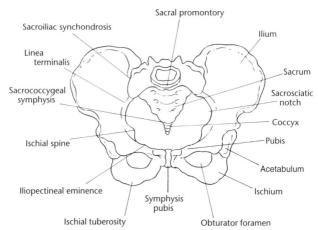

FIGURE 2-2   Bones of the Pelvis[1]

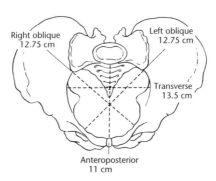

FIGURE 2-3   Diameters of the Pelvic Inlet[2]

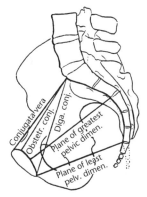

FIGURE 2-4   Pelvic Planes and Diameters
Source: Reproduced with permission from C. M. Steer. *Moloy's Evaluation of the Pelvis in Obstetrics,* 3rd ed. New York: Plenum Medical Book Company, 1975, p. 2.

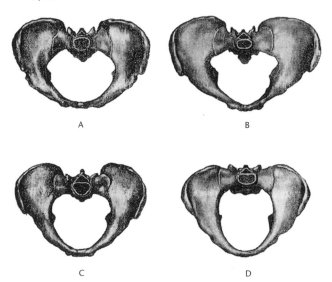

FIGURE 2-5   Types of Pelves
Caldwell-Moloy classification of female pelvis. Parent types.
A, Platypelloid; *B,* Android; *C,* Gynecoid; *D,* Anthropoid.
Source: Reproduced with permission from J. C. Ullery and M. A. Castallo. *Obstetric Mechanisms and Their Management.* Philadelphia: F. A. Davis Company, 1957, p. 39.

7

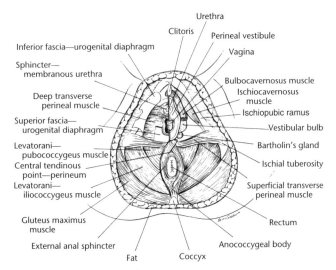

FIGURE 2-6   Perineal Anatomy
Muscles of the perineum and related structures.[3]

Fetal Skull

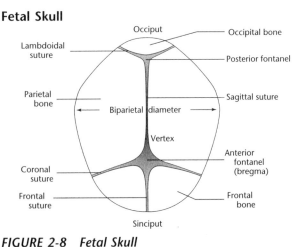

FIGURE 2-8   Fetal Skull
Landmarks, bones, fontanels, sutures, and biparietal diameter.[4]

Breast Anatomy

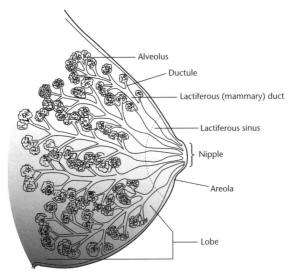

FIGURE 2-7 Anatomy of the Breast
Schematic diagram of breast.
Source: J. Riordan and K. G. Auerbach. *Breastfeeding and Human Lactation,* © 1993. Boston: Jones and Bartlett Publishers. Adapted with permission.

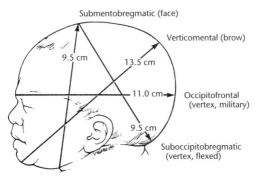

FIGURE 2-9
Possible presenting diameters of the average term fetal skull.
Source: Reproduced with permission from S. G. Gabbe, J. Niebyl, and J. L. Simpson. *Obstetrics: Normal and Problem Pregnancies,* 3rd ed. New York: Churchill Livingstone, 1996, p. 372.)

▬ Maternal Physiological Changes

Physiological Changes during First and Second Stage Labor[5]

Blood Pressure

First stage labor

- Rises during contractions, if woman is supine
  Systolic 10 to 20 mm Hg
  Diastolic 5 to 10 mm Hg
- No rise during contractions, if woman is lying on her side
- May rise with pain, fear, or apprehension
- Best taken between contractions

Second stage labor

- May rise 15 to 25 mm Hg with contractions
- May rise 10 mm Hg between contractions when woman has been pushing

Metabolism

- Aerobic and anaerobic carbohydrate metabolism steadily rise as a result of anxiety and skeletal muscle activity
- Increased metabolism causes increased body temperature, pulse, respirations, cardiac output, and fluid loss

Temperature

- Slightly elevated during labor (by 1° to 2° F or 0.5° to 1° C)
- Highest elevation during and immediately after delivery
- Elevated temperature may also indicate dehydration or infection

Pulse (cardiac rate)

- During contractions, pulse
  ↑ during increment
  ↓ during acme to rate lower than between contractions

↑ during decrement to rate usual between contractions
- Slightly higher between contractions than prelabor pulse
- ↑ during second stage, with tachycardia reaching a peak at delivery

Respirations
- Slight increase during labor
- Hyperventilation may result in alkalosis
- May be difficult to assess because of changing breathing patterns with stages of labor

Renal Changes
- Polyuria common in labor
- Evaluate the bladder for distention often
- Slight trace or increase of 1 mg/24 hours (1+) proteinuria is common
- Proteinuria of 2 mg/24 hours or more (≥2+) is not normal

Gastrointestinal Changes
- ↓ gastric motility and absorption of food
- ↓ secretion of gastric juice during labor
- ↑ gastric emptying time
- Nausea and vomiting common near end of first and beginning of second stage

Hematologic Changes
- Hemoglobin ↑ 1.2 gm/100 ml during labor
- Hemoglobin returns to prelabor levels first day postpartum if no hemorrhage occurred
- Blood coagulation time ↓
- ↑ plasma fibrinogen during labor
- White blood cell (WBC) count progressively ↑ throughout first stage by about 5000/mm^3 up to an average of 15,000/mm^3 at complete dilatation
- Blood sugar ↓ during labor; drops markedly in prolonged and difficult labors

Notes

Chapter 3

Health Care of Well Women

Health History and Examination

Routine History[1]

- Identifying information
- Chief complaint
- History of present illness
- Past medical and primary care history
- Social history
- Family history
- Menstrual history
- Obstetric history
- Gynecologic history
- Sexual history
- Contraceptive history

Routine Physical Examination and Review of Systems[2]

- Physical measurements and vital signs
- General evaluation of health status
- Skin and hair
- Head
- Eyes, ears, nose, mouth, and throat
- Neck

- Heart
- Lungs
- Breasts (see breast examination for more detail)
- Abdomen (gastrointestinal system)
- Genitourinary system
- Reproductive system (see pelvic examination for more detail)
- Musculoskeletal system
- Vascular system
- Central nervous system
- Lymphatic and hematopoietic systems

Breast Examination[3]

Relevant History

- Age
- Tumor
- Nipple discharge
- Pain or tenderness
- Past history of mammograms or breast ultrasound examinations
- Past history of breast disease
- Family history of breast disease
- Menstrual history
- Pregnancy history
- Lactation history
- Hormonal history
- Other
  Oophorectomy
  Alcohol consumption
  Radiation exposure

Physical Examination of the Breast

Inspection of breasts and nipples; palpation of breasts and lymph node areas.

Normal findings

- Breasts of unequal size but same contour
- Breasts may be small, large, or pendulous

- Accessory breast tissue—alone or any combination of supernumerary nipples, areola, glandular parenchyma
- Inverted nipples—not retracted or deviated
- No palpable nodes
- A transverse ridge, perhaps slightly tender, at the caudal edge of the breast
- Fine nodularity throughout the breast
- Coarse nodularity generalized throughout the breast, occurring during the premenstrual or menstrual phases of the menstrual cycle

Abnormal findings—physician consultation or referral required

- Asymmetry in breast contour, e.g., bulge or indentation in contour
- Retraction signs, e.g., skin dimples, puckers, furrows
- Nipple deviation or retraction, with or without broadening and flattening of the nipple
- Shrunken breast
- Edema; orange-peel skin
- Dilated subcutaneous veins in a woman who is not pregnant
- Elevation of skin temperature or redness in a woman who is not postpartal
- Ulcerations
- Excessive breast elevation and asymmetry with contraction of pectoral muscles
- Palpable nodes
- Nipple erosion, ulceration, thickening, or unusual roughness
- Nipple redness in a woman who is not breastfeeding or having nipples sexually manipulated
- Nipple crusting, indicating dried discharge in a woman who is not pregnant, postpartal, or breastfeeding

- Coarse, granular nodularity in a localized area
- Loss of elasticity of nipples or breast tissue, with increased firmness or thickening of skin texture
- Any mass; note the following:
  Location
  Size
  Shape and contour
  Consistency
  Delimitation, (degree of sharpness of the margins)
  Mobility

Contrary to popular practice, it is ***not*** necessary to attempt to express discharge from the nipples as part of a routine breast examination. Elicited discharge usually has no pathological significance. Spontaneous discharge is significant and requires physician consultation or referral.

Charting of Findings

If findings are normal: Breasts symmetrical, soft, and without masses. Nipples symmetrical, clean, and not retracted. No palpable supraclavicular or axillary nodes. History noncontributory.

If findings are abnormal:

1. Describe findings. Draw a sketch locating any mass. The sketch may be simple, simulating a clock face with the nipple in the center. Note left or right breast. Describe size, shape, consistency, delimitation, and mobility or movability of the mass.
2. Note any palpable supraclavicular or axillary nodes and the number, size, and consistency of each.
3. Describe any asymmetry or retraction signs, where located, what position the woman was in, and what maneuver elicited them.
4. Note and describe nipple changes or discharge.

5. Note relevant history.
6. End the note with the name of the physician with whom you will consult or to whom you are referring the woman.

Variations in Breast Examination and Findings for the Pregnant Woman

Because of physiological changes that occur in the breast during pregnancy, the following findings are considered normal in the pregnant woman:

1. Bilateral increase in size, often accompanied by tingling, tenseness, and tenderness.
2. Increased generalized coarse nodular and lobular feel of the breast as a result of hypertrophy of the mammary alveoli.
3. Discharge of colostrum from the nipples. May appear as early as the sixth week of gestation as a clear viscous fluid.
4. Montgomery's follicles: hypertrophied sebaceous glands in the areola.
5. Enlargement and increased erectility of the nipples.
6. Broadening and increased pigmentation of the areola.
7. Dilated subcutaneous veins, usually seen beneath the skin as a blue tracing.
8. Vascular spiders on the upper chest (also upper arms, neck, and face).
9. Striae of the breasts.

Variations in Breast Examination for the Postpartal Woman

1. Check for adequate support with a properly fitting brassiere or a breast binder.
2. Palpate the breasts to ascertain their condition
Soft
Filling—tense, increasing firmness, slightly enlarged

Engorged—enlarged, hard, reddened, shiny, painful, with skin temperature elevated, and dilated veins

3. If the mother is breastfeeding, inspect the nipple epithelium for:
Signs of irritation—reddened, tender
Precursory signs of cracking—tiny pinpoint blisters or subepithelial petechiae (best seen with a small magnifying glass)
Cracking—sore, possibly bleeding

Pelvic Examination[4]

The pelvic examination includes:

- Inspection of the external genitalia
- Examination of Bartholin's and Skene's glands and urethra (BSU)
- Speculum examination
- Bimanual examination
- Rectovaginal examination
- Clinical pelvimetry may be included as part of the bimanual examination if indicated. (See page 104.)

Types of Speculae[5]

Virginal

- Short, narrow, flat blade
- Used for young girls, women who have had little or no coitus

Graves', standard size

- 3 1/2″ long by 3/4″ wide, blades curved to form a concave space between the blades, with the posterior blade 1/4″ longer than the anterior
- Also available in plastic
- Most commonly used speculum; used for sexually active and parous women

Graves', large size

- 5″ long by 1 1/4″ wide, blades formed like standard size
- Also available in plastic
- Used for women with collapsing vaginal walls, especially grand multiparas or very obese women

Pederson

- Same length as standard Graves', but narrower, flat blades
- Used for women who may be sexually active but tight or nulliparous, or for women with vaginal senescence

Defects of Vaginal/Rectal Musculature

Urethrocele

- Bulging of distal anterior vaginal wall downward and into the introitus

Cystocele

- First degree: bulging of anterior vaginal wall; if asymptomatic, normal finding
- Second degree: bulging reaches the vaginal orifice or introitus; if asymptomatic, no treatment needed
- Third degree: bulging extends beyond the introitus

Rectocele (graded the same as cystoceles)

- Noted at the lower posterior vaginal wall by bulging up into the vagina and outward toward the introitus
- If second or third degree, ask if woman has difficulty with bowel movements

Enterocele

- Prolapse of the upper end of the posterior vaginal wall

Uterine Descensus

- First degree: any minor descent of the uterus within the vagina

- Second degree: cervix protrudes through the vaginal introitus
- Third degree: prolapse of entire uterus outside the vulva

Laboratory Tests and Adjunctive Studies for the Nonpregnant Woman

The tests and studies done as part of a routine screening vary based on the age of the woman and her risk status, e.g., if she has been exposed to sexually transmitted diseases (STDs) or tuberculosis. At a minimum, for all ages, the following laboratory tests and adjunctive studies are done at a first visit:

1. Hemoglobin/hematocrit
2. Total cholesterol
3. Urinalysis
4. Pap smear

Laboratory values for nonpregnant and pregnant women are shown in Table 3-1 on pp. 22–25.

Notes

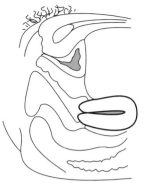

A. Midline (Military)

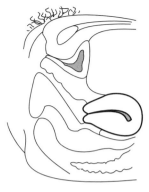

D. Retroverted

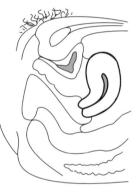

B. Anteverted

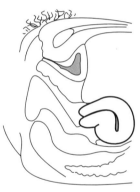

E. Retroflexed

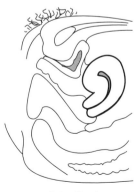

C. Anteflexed

FIGURE 3-1   Positions of the Uterus

TABLE 3-1   Table of Normal Laboratory Values for Nonpregnant and Pregnant Women

Hematology	Nonpregnant	Pregnant
Hematocrit	37%–47%	33%–44%
Hemoglobin	12.0–16.0 g/dl	10.5–14 g/dl
Erythrocyte count	$4.8 \times 10^6/mm^3$	$4.0 \times 10^6/mm^3$
Leukocyte count	$6.0(4.5–11.0) \times 10^3/mm^3$	$9.2(6–16.0) \times 10^3/mm^3$
Neutrophils	$4.4(1.8–7.7) \times 10^3/mm^3$	$(3.8–10) \times 10^3/mm^3$
Lymphocytes	$2.5(1.0–4.8) \times 10^3/mm^3$	$(1.3–5.2) \times 10^3/mm^3$
Monocytes	$0.30(0–0.8) \times 10^3/mm^3$	No change
Eosinophils	$0.20(0–0.45) \times 10^3/mm^3$	No change
Platelet count	130,000–400,000/ml	No change
Fibrinogen	200–400 ng/dl	300–600 ng/dl
Folate		
Red cell	150–450 ng/ml cells	100–400 ng/ml cells
Ferritin	15–200 ng/ml	5–150 ng/ml
Iron	135 µg/dl	90 µg/dl
Iron binding capacity	250–460 µg/dl	300–600 µg/dl
Coagulation studies		
Bleeding time (Duke)	< 4 min	No change
Partial thromboplastin time	24–36 sec	No change
Prothrombin time	12–14 sec	No change
Thrombin time	12–18 sec	No change

Factors

	Nonpregnant	Pregnant
VIII	60%–100%	120%–200%
X, IX	60%–100%	90%–120%
VII, XII	60%–100%	No change
II, V, XI	60%–100%	No change
V	60%–100%	40%–70%

Renal	Nonpregnant	Pregnant
BUN	10–20 mg/dl	5–12 mg/dl
Creatinine	<1.5 mg/dl	<1.0 mg/dl
Magnesium	2–3 mg/dl	1.6–2.1 mg/dl
Osmolality	285–295 mOsm/kg/H_2O	275–280 mOsm/kg/H_2O
Sodium	136–145 mEq/L	130–140 mEq/L
Potassium	3.5–5.0 mEq/L	3.3–4.1 mEq/L
Carbon dioxide content	21–30 mEq/L	18–25 mEq/L
Chloride	98–106 mEq/L	93–100 mEq/L
Uric acid	1.5–6.0 mg/dL	1.2–4.5 mg/dl
Urinary protein	<150 mg/day	<250–300 mg/day
Creatinine clearance	91–130 ml/min	120–160 ml/min
Complement (total)	150–250 CH50	200–400
C3	55–120 mg/dl	100–180 mg/dl

TABLE 3-1 Continued

Endocrine	Nonpregnant	Pregnant
Glucose, fasting (plasma)	75–115 mg/dl	60–105 mg/dl
ACTH	20–100 pg/ml	No change
Aldosterone (plasma)	<8 ng/dl	<20 ng/dl
Aldosterone (urinary)	8–20 μg/24 hrs	15–40 μg/24 hrs
Cortisol (plasma)	5–25 μg/dl	15–35 μg/dl
Growth hormone, fasting	<5 ng/ml	No change
Insulin, fasting	6–26 μU/ml	8–30 μU/ml
Parathyroid hormone	20–30 pg/ml	10–20 pg/ml
Prolactin	2–15 ng/ml	50–400 ng/ml
Renin activity (plasma)	0.9–3.3 ng/ml/hr	3–8 ng/ml/hr
Thyroxine, total (T_4)	5–12 μg/dl	10–17 μg/dl
Triiodothyronine (T_3)	70–190 ng/dl	100–220 ng/dl
Free T_4	1–2 ng/dl	No change
T_3 resin uptake	25%–35%	15%–25%
Free thyroxine index	1.75–4.95	No change
TSH	4–5 μU/ml	No change
Calcium		
Total	9.0–10.5 mg/dl	8.1–9.5 mg/dl
Ionized	4.5–5.6 mg/dl	4.0–5.0 mg/dl
Inorganic phosphorus	3.0–4.5 mg/dl	No change

Hepatic and Enzymes	Nonpregnant	Pregnant
Bilirubin (total)	0.3–1.0 mg/dl	No change
Cholesterol	120–180 mg/dl	180–280 mg/dl
Triglyceride	<160 mg/dl	<260 mg/dl
Amylase	60–180 U/L	90–350 U/L
Creatine phosphokinase	10–70 U/L	5–40 U/L
Lactic dehydrogenase (LDH)	200–450 Units/ml	No change
Lipase	4–24 IU/dl	2–12 IU/dl
Alkaline phosphatase	30–95 mU/ml	60–200 mU/ml
Alanine amino transaminase (SGPT)	0–35 U/L	No change
Aspartate amino transaminase (SGOT)	0–35 U/L	No change
Gamma-glutamyl transpeptidase	1–45 IU/L	No change
Ceruloplasmin	27–37 mg/dl	40–60 mg/dl
Copper	70–140 ng/dl	120–200 ng/dl
Protein (total)	5.5–8.0 g/dl	4.5–7.0 g/dl
Albumin	3.5–5.5 g/dl	2.5–4.5 g/dl
IgA	90–325 mg/dl	No change
IgM	45–150 mg/dl	No change
IgG	800–1,500 mg/dl	700–1400 mg/dl

Source: G. N. Burrows and T. F. Ferris. *Medical Complications During Pregnancy,* 4th ed. Philadelphia: W. B. Saunders Company, 1995, inside front and back covers.

Family Planning Method Effectiveness

TABLE 3-2 *Percentage of Women Experiencing a Contraceptive Failure During the First Year of Typical Use and the First Year of Perfect Use and Percentage Continuing Use at the End of the First Year, United States*[6]

Method	% Experiencing an Accidental Pregnancy within the First Year of Use		% Continuing Use at 1 Year[3]
	Typical use[1]	Perfect use[2]	
Chance[4]	85	85	
Spermicides[5]	21	6	43
Periodic abstinence	20		67
Calendar		9	
Ovulation method		3	
Sympto-thermal[6]		2	
Post-ovulation		1	
Withdrawal	19	4	
Cap[7]			
Parous women	36	26	45
Nulliparous women	18	9	58
Sponge			
Parous women	36	20	45
Nulliparous women	18	9	58
Diaphragm[7]	18	6	58
Condom[8]			
Female	21	5	56
Male	12	3	63
Pill	3		72
Progestin only		0.5	
Combined		0.1	
Intrauterine device (IUD)			
Progesterone T	2.0	1.5	81
Copper T 380A	0.8	0.6	78
LNG-20	0.1	0.1	81
Depo-Provera	0.3	0.3	70
Norplant (6 capsules)	0.09	0.09	85
Female sterilization	0.4	0.4	100
Male sterilization	0.15	0.10	100

TABLE 3-2 Notes

Emergency contraceptive pills: Treatment initiated within 72 hr after unprotected intercourse reduces the risk of pregnancy by at least 75%.[9]

Lactational amenorrhea method (LAM): is a highly effective, *temporary* method of contraception.[10]

[1] Among *typical* couples who initiate use of a method (not necessarily for the first time), the percentage who experience an accidental pregnancy during the first year if they do not stop use for any other reason

[2] Among couples who initiate use of a method (not necessarily for the first time) and who use it *perfectly* (both consistently and correctly), the percentage who experience an accidental pregnancy during the first year if they do not stop use for any other reason

[3] Among couples attempting to avoid pregnancy, the percentage who continue to use a method for one year

[4] The percentages failing in columns (2) and (3) are based on data from populations where contraception is not used and from women who cease using contraception in order to become pregnant. Among such populations, about 89% become pregnant within 1 year. This estimate was lowered slightly (to 85%) to represent the percentage who would become pregnant within 1 year among women now relying on reversible methods of contraception if they abandoned contraception altogether.

[5] Foams, creams, gels, vaginal suppositories, and vaginal film

[6] Cervical mucus (ovulation) method supplemented by calendar in the preovulatory and basal body temperature in the postovulatory phases

[7] With spermicidal cream or jelly

[8] Without spermicides

[9] The treatment schedule is one dose as soon as possible (but no more than 72 hr) after unprotected intercourse, and a second dose 12 hr after the first dose. The hormones that have been studied in the clinical trials of postcoital hormonal contraception are found in Nordette, Levlen, Lo/Ovral (1 dose is 4 pills), Triphasil, Tri-Levlen (1 dose is 4 yellow pills), and Ovral (1 dose is 2 pills).

[10] However, to maintain effective protection against pregnancy, another method of contraception must be used as soon as menstruation resumes, the frequency or duration of breastfeeds is reduced, bottle feeds are introduced, or the baby reaches 6 months of age.

Source: Reprinted with permission of R. A. Hatcher et al. *Contraceptive Technology,* 16th rev ed New York, Irvington Publishers, Inc., 1991, pp. 113–114.

Intrauterine Contraceptive Devices (IUDs)[7]

Types of IUDs
- Copper T 380A (ParaGard)
- Progesterone T (Progestasert)
- Levonorgestrel IUD (LNG-20)

Absolute Contraindications

- Pregnancy—known or suspected
- Pelvic inflammatory disease (PID)—history or current
- Cervical or uterine carcinoma—known or suspected
  Unresolved, abnormal Pap smears (class III, CIN 1, or greater)
  Unexplained or abnormal uterine bleeding
- History or presence of valvular heart disease (not including mitral valve prolapse)
- Presence of myomata, congenital malformations, or developmental anomalies that distort the uterine cavity
- Known or suspected allergy to copper or Wilson's disease (only for IUDs with copper)
- Uterine sound measurements outside the limits stated in the most recent insertion instructions from the manufacturer
- High risk for STDs
- History of or high risk for ectopic pregnancy—only contraindicated for Progestasert
- Acute cervicitis (until diagnosed and treated)
- Genital actinomycosis
- Increased susceptibility to infection, e.g., chronic corticosteroid therapy, diabetes, blood dyscrasias, human immunodeficiency virus (HIV) infection

Relative Contraindications

- History of dysmenorrhea
- History of menorrhagia
- History of metrorrhagia
- Nulliparity
- History of previous unsuccessful use or problems with an IUD
- History of severe vasovagal response

Safety Measures for IUD Insertion

- Careful selection of the woman to rule out contraindications
- Use of sterile instruments, including the speculum
- Strict adherence to sterile technique throughout the procedure
- Thorough cleansing of the cervix with an antiseptic agent
- Careful bimanual examination to determine the position of the uterus
- Proper application and use of the tenaculum on the cervix
- Careful sounding of the uterus and measurement of its depth
- Fundal placement of the IUD
- Slow and gentle pace
- Read the manufacturer's instructions for details pertaining to the specific IUD

Management of Syncope

- Use Trendelenburg position
- Maintain open airway
- Keep woman warm
- Use aromatics (smelling salts)
- If severe, administer 0.4 to 0.5 mg atropine IM

Signs and symptoms of PID

See page 75.

Pregnancy with an IUD in Place

Risks include:

- Intrauterine infections
- Sepsis
- Spontaneous abortion
- Septic abortion
- Ectopic pregnancy
- Preterm labor
- Placenta previa

If the strings of the IUD are visible, remove the IUD: 25% of women will abort spontaneously; 50% will lose the pregnancy if the IUD is left in place. Removal avoids the risk of spontaneous septic abortion while waiting for a therapeutic pregnancy termination and decreases the risks listed above.

If the strings are not visible or accessible in the cervix, obtain an ultrasound examination to determine whether the IUD has been expelled. If the IUD is still present, the woman should be offered the option of a therapeutic abortion.

Oral Hormonal Contraception[8]

Noncontraceptive Benefits
- Reduction in ovarian cancer
- Reduction in endometrial cancer
- Decreased dysmenorrhea
- Reduction of hirsutism
- Reduction of acne
- Decreased blood loss during menses, leading to decreased anemia and increased iron stores
- Decreased benign breast disease
- Protection against and treatment for endometriosis

Absolute Contraindications
- Pregnancy—known or suspected
- Thrombophlebitis (presence or history)
- Thromboembolic disorders (presence or history)
- Cerebrovascular accident (presence or history)
- Cerebrovascular disease (presence or history)
- Coronary occlusion or heart attack (presence or history)
- Liver damage, impaired liver function, or acute hepatitis
- Benign or malignant liver tumor (presence or history)
- Estrogen-dependent neoplasia (presence or history)

- Undiagnosed abnormal genital bleeding
- Carcinoma of the reproductive system (presence or history)
- Classic migraine headaches (with aura)

Relative Contraindications

Use extreme caution, consult, and make individualized decisions for women with these clinical situations.

- Smoking over age 35
- Hypertension (blood pressure $\geq$ 140/90)
- Diabetes mellitus
- Asthma
- Cardiac disease (presence or history)
- Renal disease (presence or history)
- Gallbladder disease (presence or history)
- Lupus erythematosus
- Depression (presence or history)
- Elective surgery requiring lengthy immobilization
- Over 50 years of age
- Carcinoma of the breast—known or suspected*

*Risk determined by hormone receptor status.

Side Effects and Complications

See Table 3-3 on page 32.

Notes

TABLE 3-3   Relation of Side Effects to Hormone Content [9]

Hormone Status	Reproductive System	Premenstrual Syndrome	General	Cardiovascular System
Estrogen excess	Breast cystic changes Cervical extrophy Dysmenorrhea Hypermenorrhea, menorrhagia, and clotting Increase in breast size Mucorrhea Uterine enlargement Uterine fibroid growth	Bloating Dizziness, syncope Edema Headache (cyclic) Irritability Leg cramps Nausea, vomiting Visual changes (cyclic) Weight gain (cyclic)	Chloasma Chronic nasal pharyngitis Gastric influenza and varicella Hay fever and allergic rhinitis Urinary tract infection	Capillary fragility Cerebrovascular accident Deep vein thrombosis Hemiparesis (unilateral weakness and numbness) Telangiectasias Thromboembolic disease
Estrogen deficiency	Absence of withdrawal bleeding Atrophic vaginitis Bleeding and spotting during pill days 1 to 9 Continuous bleeding and spotting Flow decrease, hypomenorrhea Pelvic relaxation symptoms		Nervousness Vasomotor symptoms	

Progestin excess	Cervicitis Decrease in flow length Moniliasis	Appetite increase Depression Fatigue Hypoglycemia symptoms Libido decrease Neurodermatitis Weight gain (non-cyclic)	Hypertension Leg vein dilation
Progestin deficiency	Breakthrough bleeding and spotting during pill days 10 to 21 Delayed withdrawal bleeding Dysmenorrhea Heavy flow and clots, hypermenorrhea, menorrhagia		
Androgen excess		Acne Cholestatic jaundice Hirsutism Libido increase Oily skin and scalp Rash and pruritus Edema	

Source: Adapted with permission from R. P. Dickey. *Managing Contraceptive Pill Patients,* 8th ed. Durant, Oklahoma: Essential Medical Information Systems, 1994, Table 11, pp. 148–149. Used with permission.

TABLE 3-4   *Oral Contraceptive (OC) Interactions with Selected Medications*

Action of Medication	Recommendation
Reduced effectiveness of OCs	
Rifampin (Rifamycin, Rifadin; antituberculosis med)	Women should choose another contraceptive method
Phenytoin (Dilantin; antiseizure med) Primidone (Mysoline; antiseizure med) Carbamazepine (Tegretol; antiseizure med) Phenobarbital (Donnatol, antispasmodic/sedative) Griseofulvin (Fulvicin; antifungal trt)	If OCs are strongly indicated, a higher dose of estrogen may be used with antiseizure meds
Tetracycline Penicillin	Use alternate/additional contraceptive during course of therapy, such as condoms; not necessary to discontinue use of OCs
Potentiation of OCs	
Vitamin C, > 1 g/day	Increases ethinyl estradiol by 50%; decrease Vit C to 1000 mg/day
Action potentiated by OCs	
Diazepam (Valium; antianxiety med) Benzodiazepine tranquilizers (Librium, Ativan,	Use medication with caution; greatest impairment during menstrual pause in OC use

Serax, Tranxene, Xanax; antianxiety/sedative)	
Theophylline (Aerolate, Bronkotabs, Marax, Respbid, Theolair; bronchodilators for asthma)	Monitor theophyline concentration
Tricyclic antidepressants (Tofranil, Elavil, Norpramin)	Monitor antidepressant action
Corticosteroids/cortisone (Cortone; antiinflammatory)	Clinical significance not established
Beta-blockers (Corgard, Inderal, Lopressor, Tenormin)	Monitor cardiovascular status
Alcohol	Use alcohol with caution
Effectiveness reduced by OCs	
Guanethidine (Ismelin, Esimel; antihypertensive)	Use alternate contraceptive
Methyldopa (Aldoclor, Aldomet, Aldoril; antihypertensive	
Anticoagulants (oral)	
Hypoglycemics (Tolbutamide, Diabinese, Orinase, Tolinase)	Monitor blood glucose
Acetaminophen (Tylenol; analgesic)	Monitor pain-relieving response

Warning Symptoms of Adverse Reactions to Oral Contraceptives

Discontinue oral contraceptives and initiate physician consultation.

- Headaches—severe, persistent, of sudden onset, or qualitatively different from those a woman normally experiences
- Visual disturbances
  Blurring of vision
  Flashing lights
  Diplopia
  Scintillating scotomata
  Periods of temporary blindness
- Unexplained severe chest pain or shortness of breath
- Unexplained severe abdominal pain
- Severe calf or thigh pain
- Temporary numbness or paralysis of any part of the face or body
- Slurring of speech
- Hemoptysis
- Marked increase in blood pressure

The woman should be provided with another method of family planning when she must stop taking the pill because of side effects, complications, or undesirable drug interactions.

Principles of Pill Switching

- If switching to an equal or greater dose of estrogen/progestin, switch any time in cycle
- If switching to less estrogen/progestin, switch at beginning of new cycle
- If woman is confused about pill cycles, switch at beginning of new cycle

Long-Term Hormonal Contraception[10]

Depo-Provera

Absolute contraindications

1. Pregnancy—known or suspected
2. History of breast cancer
3. Genital bleeding of unknown origin

Relative contraindications

1. History of depression
2. History of any kind of breast disease
3. History of migraine headaches
4. The woman's desire to become pregnant within the next year or two
5. The woman's desire to time a pregnancy within a rather narrow time range

Selection

1. Adolescents to women in their 40s
2. Nulligravidas to grand multiparas
3. Women who are breastfeeding (after 6 weeks postpartum)
4. Women with liver disease* (despite what the package insert says)
5. Women with hemoglobinopathy
6. Women with hypertension
7. Women with a history of thromboembolism‖ (despite what the package insert says)
8. Women with seizure disorders
9. Women over age 35 who smoke
10. Women for whom estrogen is contraindicated

*‖A. M. Kaunitz, DMPA: A new contraceptive option. *Contemporary OB/GYN,* 19–34 (January) 1993.

Side effects that affect all women on Depo-Provera

1. Menstrual changes—unpredictable irregular bleeding and spotting for several months until amenorrhea ensues in most women

2. Delayed return of fertility after discontinuation—50%–70% of women conceive by end of 1 year but delay may be as long as 18–24 months

Benefits

1. Improves certain medical conditions
   Anemia (increases hemoglobin because of reduced menses)
   Decreased risk of ascending infection or PID
   Decreased frequency of sickle cell disease crises with increased red blood cell survival
   Menorrhagia
   Decreased frequency of seizures in seizure disorders
2. Does not interact with other drugs to the detriment of contraceptive efficacy
3. Associated with the prevention of endometrial cancer

Management of care

1. Pre-method counseling about side effects and delay in return to fertility
2. Monitoring for breast cancer
   Teach monthly breast self-examination
   Annual breast examination performed by a health care professional
   Baseline mammogram, if woman has a personal or family history of breast disease
3. Postpartum use
   If bottle-feeding, initiate within 5 days of delivery
   If breastfeeding, initiate at 6 weeks postpartum after milk supply is well established (small amounts of Depo-Provera found in breast milk are not detrimental to either the breast milk or the baby)

4. Importance of returning for injection every 12 weeks
5. Use of condoms, if at risk for HIV or STD

Norplant (levonorgestrel)

Absolute contraindications

1. Pregnancy—known or suspected
2. Abnormal genital bleeding of unknown origin
3. Active thrombophlebitis or thromboembolism disorders
4. Acute disease of the liver; benign or malignant liver tumors
5. Known or suspected breast cancer

The contraceptive effectiveness of levonorgestrel is compromised when the woman is taking drugs for the treatment of tuberculosis (e.g., Rifampin) or seizure activity (e.g., Dilantin). Such women should use a backup contraceptive method while on these drugs and for 2 weeks after completing drug therapy.

Selection

Women for whom Norplant would be an appropriate choice include the following.

1. Women who are breastfeeding (after 6 weeks postpartum)
2. Women who have had unacceptable side effects from oral contraceptive pills containing estrogen
3. Women who have difficulty remembering to take a pill or an aversion to the manipulation needed for the barrier methods
4. Women who want long-term contraception (e.g., women who are finished with childbearing but don't want sterilization)
5. Women who want to be able to time a pregnancy

Major side effects

1. Irregular menstrual bleeding, ranging from amenorrhea to prolonged bleeding
2. Headaches

Management of care

1. Pre-method counseling about side effects
2. Insertion within 7 days of the start of a menstrual period
3. Postpartum insertion
   Immediately postabortion or postpartum if not breastfeeding
   6 weeks postpartum if breastfeeding

4. Use of condoms, if at risk for HIV or STD

Emergency Postcoital Contraception[11]

Should be considered for any woman who has had unprotected intercourse within the last 72 hours and does not wish to be pregnant. Circumstances for such women include:

- A woman who has been raped or sexually assaulted
- Intercourse without contraception
- Multiple oral contraceptive pills have been missed (3 or more midcycle or any 7 days without pills)
- One or more progestin-only pills have been missed
- A barrier method has been used incorrectly, was dislodged, or was removed too early
- A condom broke, slipped, or leaked
- Withdrawal or periodic abstinence has been unsuccessful
- Ejaculation on the external genitalia has occurred
- An IUD has been partially or completely expelled
- When an IUD is necessarily removed midcycle
- When there has been exposure to possible teratogen, e.g., live vaccine, cytotoxic drug, extensive X-ray studies

Considerations for Determining
Postcoital Treatment

- Would short-term, high-dose estrogen and progestin create undue health risks?
- Are danazol, progestin-only pills, or an IUD better options than high-dose combination oral contraceptive pills for this woman?
- Would the woman elect to terminate the pregnancy if she became pregnant?

Contraindications

To oral contraceptives (high-dose estrogen and progestin or progestins only)
- Same as for any use of OCs

To use of danazol
- Abnormal vaginal bleeding of unknown origin
- Impaired liver, kidney, or heart function
- Porphyria
- Intention to continue pregnancy if emergency postcoital contraception fails (may cause androgenic effects on a female fetus)
- Breastfeeding

To IUD
- Same as for any woman using an IUD

Side Effects

Oral contraceptives (high-dose estrogen and progestin
- Nausea—occurs in 50% to 70% of women
- Vomiting—occurs in 25% of women
- Breast tenderness
- Dizziness
- Headache
- Abdominal pain

Progestin-only oral contraceptives and danazol
- Same as above, but occur less often

- Menstrual cycle disturbances with abnormal bleeding; the next menses may come several days sooner or later than anticipated; **if no menses occur within 3 weeks, evaluate for pregnancy**

Management of Emergency Contraception

If treatment cannot be arranged by phone, an emergency visit must be scheduled or the woman must be referred to an available source.

History
- Past medical history
- Menstrual history
  Last menstrual period (LMP), previous menses
  Usual menstrual pattern
  Estimated date of ovulation
- History of coitus—date and number of hours since the first and most recent unprotected episodes
- Contraceptive history
  Any current contraceptive use?
  Type of contraceptives used
- Contraindications to oral contraceptives and IUDs

Management Actions
- Compare possible ovulation with timing of unprotected intercourse to elaluate risk of pregnancy
- Determine woman's concerns about possible pregnancy and if she is a candidate for emergency post-coital contraception
- Determine if additional physical, pelvic, and laboratory tests are indicated
- Discuss options with the woman
- Plan for interim and ongoing contraception
- Prescribe emergency contraception (see Table 3-5)
- Plan for follow-up care; **if menses have not occurred within 3 weeks, must evaluate for pregnancy**

Managing Side Effects

Treatment of nausea
- If patient vomits soon after taking a dose, she may

TABLE 3-5 **Emergency Contraception Dosages**

Drug	Dosage	Frequency
Ovral	2 pills	2 doses, 12 hr apart
Lo/Ovral, Nordette, Levlen	4 pills	2 doses, 12 hr apart
Triphasil, Tri-Levlen	4 yellow pills	2 doses, 12 hr apart
Ovrette (progestin only)	16 pills	Single dose within 8–12 hr after intercourse
Danazol	400 mg po	3 doses, 12 hr apart

It is generally necessary to prescribe one full pack of pills, because they are not packaged in the above quantities. Women should be instructed to take only the prescribed number of pills—a higher dose will not minimize the risk of pregnancy, but will probably increase side effects.

need replacement medication; some providers prescribe extra pills to use in case of vomiting
- Dramamine (dimenhydrinate) 50 mg one or two tabs po q 4–6 hr (may take dose 30 min before taking pills)
- Marezine (cyclizine hydrochloride) 50 mg po q 4–6 hr
- Tigan (trimethobenzamide HCl) 250 mg po q 8 hr, or 200 mg rectal suppository q 8 hr
- Phenergan (promethazine HCl) 25 mg po q 12 hr, or 25 mg rectal suppository q 12 hr

If the woman has severe abdominal pain, or heavy vaginal bleeding, an examination is indicated.

Intrauterine Contraceptive Device
- Can be inserted within 5 to 7 days after unprotected intercourse
- Perform pregnancy test first
- Not a good method for rape victims because of potential for STDs and infection

Notes

▭ Care of Perimenopausal Women

Perimenopausal Visit[12]

Perimenopausal History

In addition to the routine history, obtain information on perimenopausal changes and specific risk factors associated with

- Reproductive tract
- Urinary tract
- Breasts
- Vasomotor system (hot flushes, night sweats)
- Skeletal system
- Cardiovascular system
- Psychological changes

The following symptoms of estrogen excess may present in perimenopausal women

- Uterine bleeding
- Bloating
- Growth of uterine fibroids
- Endometriosis

Assessment of the midlife woman should also focus on early detection of any of the major chronic diseases

- Hypertension
- Heart disease
- Diabetes mellitus
- Cancer

Each of the following should be investigated before completing a management plan

- Impairments of vision
- Impairments of hearing
- Dental health
- Nutritional status
- Physical activities or limitations

- Injury prevention (seat belt use, avoidance of drinking and driving)
- Environmental risks
- Occupational, sexual, marital, relationship, and parental problems
- Use of cigarettes, alcohol, and other substances
- Contraceptive needs
- Immunization status

Perimenopausal Physical Examination[13]

The annual examination should include items of importance to the woman who is in the climacteric

1. Height: women may have lost an inch or more. Measuring height provides an opportunity to discuss posture, body mechanics, exercise, and osteoporosis.
2. Skin: evaluate for integrity, lesions, and changes in moles.
3. Mouth, teeth, gums
4. Pelvic examination: with attention to the changes that accompany aging; a Pederson speculum may be optimal for postmenopausal women.
5. Rectum: examine for occult blood, masses, and fissures.

Perimenopausal Laboratory Tests and Adjunctive Studies

Tests for routine screening, initial examinations, or annual examinations[14]

- Urinalysis/urine dipstick
- Pap smear (hormonal maturation index or cornification count optional)
- Mammography, yearly between ages 50 and 70 (thereafter mammography is probably not cost-effective)
- Stool for guaiac (occult blood)
- Fasting plasma cholesterol and triglyceride levels

and lipid profile, every 3 to 5 years if normal
- Hemoglobin/hematocrit
- Proctosigmoidoscopy, every 3 to 5 years beginning at age 50

Optional tests and adjunctive studies to be used based on clinical profile, individual risk factors, cost-effectiveness, and site policies

- Maturation index
- Cornification count
- Pituitary gonadotropins: FSH, LH
- Estrogen levels
- Fasting and 2-hour postprandial glucose levels
- Liver function tests
- Thyroid function tests
- Endometrial biopsy
- Pelvic ultrasonography
- X-ray measurement of bone mass (bone densitometry)

Hormone Replacement Therapy (HRT)

Candidates for HRT include women who have unacceptable menopausal symptoms, those who undergo early surgical menopause, and those who desire long-term prophylaxis with hormone therapy. Options such as lifestyle changes, herbal remedies, and other therapies, which may reduce the risks of cardiovascular disease and osteoporosis, should also be offered.

Goals of care include
- Relief for short-term physical and psychosocial changes
- Protection against osteoporosis
- Protection against cardiovascular disease

Keys to successful therapy
1. Women with an intact uterus need both estrogen and progesterone.
2. Women may respond best to different formulas.

3. Counseling includes side effects, risks/benefits, rationale for long-term use, alternatives, and contraindications.
4. Women with abnormal vaginal bleeding need prompt evaluation.

Decision-making for HRT*

Assist women in determining

1. The degree of disability caused by existing symptoms
2. Their desire for symptom relief
3. Their philosophy and beliefs regarding exogenous hormones
4. Their individual risks for osteoporosis, cardiovascular disease, and breast cancer, based on family and personal history, gynecologic history, physical characteristics, medical and medication history, and the practice of risk reduction or risk-enhancing behaviors
5. Their previous experience with medication compliance
6. Their previous experience with alternative treatments
7. Their willingness to use alternative treatments, such as herbs, exercise, and diet or dietary supplementation
8. Their willingness to modify or eliminate detrimental behaviors (such as poor diet, smoking, and alcohol use)
9. Their personal fears and attitudes toward aging and toward various diseases

For some women, economic considerations may enter into their decision; for others, the wishes of family members may be important.

Source: American College of Nursing-Midwives. Reprinted with permission. R. Lichtman. Perimenopausal and postmenopausal hormone replacement therapy. Part 1. An update of the literature on benefits and risks. *JNM* 41(1): 3–24, January/February, 1996, p. 22.

Contraindications
- History of thromboembolus or thrombosis
- Estrogen-dependent tumors
- Impaired liver function
- Hypertension and abnormal vaginal bleeding should be evaluated before beginning HRT but may not contraindicate its use
- A history of endometrial or breast cancer requires physician evaluation for acceptability of HRT

Common side effects
- Nausea
- Headache
- Breakthrough bleeding
- Depression
- Emotional changes
- Breast tenderness
- Bloating
- Continuation of menstrual cycle
- Failure to relieve symptoms

Notes

TABLE 3-6 Commonly Prescribed HRT Regimens

Regimen	Hormone	Dose	Taken	Advantages	Disadvantages
Sequential estrogen and progestin	Estrogen		Days 1–25 of month	Mostly widely studied in U.S. (especially with conjugated estrogen and MPA*)	Cyclic withdrawal bleeding; progestin may be difficult to tolerate
	Conjugated estrogen	0.625 mg			
	Estropipate	0.625 mg			
	Esterified estrogen	0.625 mg			
	Micronized estradiol	1 mg			
	Transdermal estrogen	0.05 mg			
	Progestin		Days 14–25 or 16–25 of month		
	MPA	10 mg			
Continuous estrogen and progestin	Estrogen		Every day	No withdrawal bleeding; easy-to-follow regimen; lower dose of progestin may increase tolerance	Erratic bleeding at start of therapy
	Conjugated estrogen	0.625 mg			
	Estropipate	0.625 mg			
	Esterified estrogen	0.625 mg			
	Micronized estradiol	1 mg			
	Transdermal estrogen	0.05 mg			
	Progestin		Every day		
	MPA	2.5–5 mg			

Continuous estrogen and cyclic progestin	Estrogen			Easy-to-follow regimen; therapy never discontinued; may be easier to assess abnormal bleeding	Cyclic withdrawal bleeding; progestin may be difficult to tolerate
	Conjugated estrogen	0.625 mg	Every day		
	Estropipate	0.625 mg			
	Esterified estrogen	0.625 mg			
	Micronized estradiol	1 mg			
	Transdermal estrogen	0.05 mg			
	Progestin				
	MPA	10 mg	Days 1–10 or 1–12 of calendar month		

*Medroxy-progesterone acetate

Source: American College of Nurse-Midwives. Reprinted with permission. R. Lichtman. Perimenopausal and postmenopausal hormone replacement therapy. Part 2. Hormonal regimens and complementary and alternative therapies. *JNM* 41(3): 195–210, 1996, p. 200.

Osteoporosis Prevention and Therapy

- Weight bearing exercise for 30 minutes 3 times per week (e.g., walking 1-1/2 miles, calisthenics) increases bone mineral content
- Estrogen preparations
  Conjugated equine estrogen (Premarin) 0.625 mg/day
  Micronized estradiol (Estrace) 0.5 mg/day
  Estropipate (Ogen, Ortho-Est) 1.25 mg/day
  Transdermal estrogen (Estraderm, Climara) 0.05 mg/day
- Calcium and vitamin supplements (to be used with or without estrogen replacement therapy [ERT])
  Calcium 1000 mg po daily for women using ERT
  Calcium 1500 mg po daily for women not using ERT
  Vitamin D 400 to 800 IU daily
- Osteoporosis prevention agents (may also be used by women *not* taking ERT)
  Calcitonin-salmon (Miacalcin nasal spray), 200 IU/day in a single puff; used in combination with calcium and vitamin D
  Alendronate (Fosamax), 10 mg po, taken on arising, with a full glass of water, 30 minutes before eating

Chapter 4

Common Health Problems

Screening for Alcohol Abuse[1]

A useful tool for obtaining an accurate alcohol history is T-ACE*, four simple questions that can be asked as part of the health history to identify women abusing alcohol.

T   How many drinks does it Take to make you feel high? (tolerance)

A   Have people Annoyed you by criticizing your drinking?

C   Have you felt you ought to Cut down on your drinking?

E   Have you ever had a drink first thing in the morning to steady your nerves or get rid of a hangover (Eye opener)?

*R.A. Welch and R.J. Sokol. Detecting risk drinking. *Contemporary OB/GYN* 36(4): 44 (April) 1991.

Tolerance is demonstrated when the woman answers "four or five drinks" or "a six-pack" or "I can drink all night and not be drunk." An affirmative answer to any of the remaining questions is also correlated with risk levels of alcohol consumption.*

*R.S. Sokol, S.I. Miller, and S. Martier. *Identifying the Alcohol-Abusing Obstetric/Gynecologic Patient: A Practical Approach.* DHHS Publication No. (ADM) 81–1163. Washington, DC: USDHHS, National Institute on Alcohol Abuse and Alcoholism, 1981.

Screening for Depression

Criteria for Major Depressive Episode[||]

A. Five (or more) of the following symptoms have been present during the same 2-week period and represent a change from previous functioning; at least one of the symptoms is either (1) depressed mood or (2) loss of interest or pleasure. *Note:* Do not include symptoms that are clearly due to a general medical condition, or mood-incongruent delusions or hallucinations.

1. Depressed mood most of the day, nearly every day, as indicated by either subjective report (e.g., feels sad or empty) or observation made by others (e.g., appears tearful). *Note:* In children and adolescents, can be irritable mood.

2. Markedly diminished interest or pleasure in all, or almost all, activities most of the day, nearly every day (as indicated by either subjective account or observation made by others)

3. Significant weight loss when not dieting or weight gain (e.g., a change of more than 5% of body weight in a month), or decrease or increase in appetite nearly every day. *Note:* In children, consider failure to make expected weight gains.

4. Insomnia or hypersomnia nearly every day

5. Psychomotor agitation or retardation nearly every day (observable by others, not merely subjective feelings of restlessness or being slowed down)

6. Fatigue or loss of energy nearly every day

7. Feelings of worthlessness or excessive or inappropriate guilt (which may be delusional) nearly every day (not merely self-reproach or guilt about being sick)

8. Diminished ability to think or concentrate, or indecisiveness, nearly every day (either by subjective account or as observed by others)

9. Recurrent thoughts of death (not just fear of dying), recurrent suicidal ideation without a specific plan, or a suicide attempt or a specific plan for committing suicide

B. The symptoms do not meet criteria for a Mixed Episode.

C. The symptoms cause clinically significant distress or impairment in social, occupational, or other important areas of functioning.

D. The symptoms are not due to the direct physiological effects of a substance (e.g., a drug of abuse, a medication) or a general medical condition (e.g., hypothyroidism).

E. The symptoms are not better accounted for by Bereavement, i.e., after the loss of a loved one, the symptoms persist for longer than 2 months or are characterized by marked functional impairment, morbid preoccupation with worthlessness, suicidal ideation, psychotic symptoms, or psychomotor retardation.

‖American Psychiatric Association: *Diagnostic and Statistical Manual of Mental Disorders,* 4th ed. Washington, DC, American Psychiatric Association, 1994. Reprinted with permission from the *Diagnostic and Statistical Manual of Mental Disorders,* 4th ed. Copyright © 1994 American Psychiatric Association.

Management of Pap Smear Results

TABLE 4-1 Reporting Classifications for Pap Smear Results and Subsequent Midwifery Management[2]

Papanicolaou Classification	CIN* Classification	The Bethesda System	Interpretation	Management
Class I	Normal	Within normal limits	Normal; no or minimal inflammatory changes	Schedule next screening Pap smear
Class II: atypical; inflammatory		Benign cellular changes; reactive and reparative changes	Inflammatory changes	Treat any vaginitis/cervicitis or STD; decrease risk factors; promote condom use; refer
		Atypical squamous or glandular cells of undetermined significance	May be either reactive changes or the start of a premalignant/ malignant process	woman to smoking cessation program; repeat Pap in 3 months; if no change in repeat Pap, refer for colposcopy

Class III	CIN-I	Low-grade SIL[||]; mild dysplasia	HPV infection	Refer for colposcopy and further evaluation, diagnosis, and treatment by physician
	CIN-II	High-grade SIL; moderate dysplasia		Refer to gynecologist/oncologist
Class IV	CIN-III	High-grade SIL; severe dysplasia; cancer in situ		Refer to gynecologist/oncologist
Class V	Invasive	Squamous cell carcinoma; adenocarcinoma	Malignant changes	Refer to gynecologist/oncologist

*CIN = cervical intraepithelial neoplasia
[||]SIL = squamous intraepithelial lesion

Screening of Women with Intrauterine Exposure to Diethylstilbestrol (DES)[3]

DES was widely used to prevent a number of complications of pregnancy from 1948 to 1971, until the FDA withdrew approval for its use in pregnancy because of association with clear cell adenocarcinoma in women exposed to DES in utero ("DES daughters"). Most clear cell adenocarcinomas in DES daughters have occurred before age 30. Other structural and functional abnormalities have also been identified as effects of in-utero exposure to DES. In 1995, the majority of exposed women were between the ages of 24 and 47.

Women exposed to DES in utero should have:

1. Their first Pap smear at menarche, age 14, or initiation of sexual intercourse, whichever comes first
2. Baseline colposcopy considered
3. Vaginal and cervical Pap smears every 6 to 12 months until age 30
4. Vaginal and cervical Pap smears every year after age 30
5. A referral for colposcopy for any abnormal spotting or bleeding

Symptoms and Prevention of Toxic Shock Syndrome[4]

Symptoms (onset sudden and severe)
- High fever (102°F or higher)
- Vomiting
- Copious watery diarrhea
- Dizziness
- Fainting or feeling faint when standing
- Sore throat
- Headache
- Severe myalgia
- Bloodshot eyes

- Hypotensive shock occurs within 48 hours and includes
  Oliguria
  Disorientation
  Combativeness
  Diffuse erythematous rash (sunburn-like)
- Laboratory test results are negative for blood, throat, and cerebrospinal fluid cultures

Possible Sequelae without Treatment
- Cardiac dysfunction
- Respiratory distress
- Death

Possible Long-term Sequelae with Treatment
- Cold and cyanotic extremities
- Weakness and fatigue associated with myopathy
- Carpal and tarsal tunnel syndromes
- Loss of mental acuity

Prevention Counseling
- Do not use high-absorbency tampons
- Alternate tampons and sanitary pads
- Do not use tampons at night
- Do not use tampons during the postpartum period

Differential Diagnosis of Dysfunctional Uterine Bleeding (DUB)

DUB is irregular vaginal bleeding caused by anovulatory menstrual cycles in the absence of illness or pathology. DUB produces episodes of heavy, prolonged bleeding and irregular cycles, sometimes to the point of amenorrhea.

Differential Diagnosis
- Pregnancy-related bleeding (e.g., spontaneous abortion, ectopic pregnancy)
- Vaginitis/cervicitis
- Effects of medications (e.g., ginseng)

- Foreign body (e.g., tampon)
- Hormonal contraception
- Endometrial hyperplasia
- Fibroids
- Cervical polyps
- Endometrial cancer
- Cervical cancer
- Thyroid disease
- Coagulation disorders
- Endometriosis

Amenorrhea Workup

Primary Amenorrhea

Defined as the absence of menstruation by age 16, or by age 14 if there have been no secondary sexual changes or growth. Refer to a gynecologist or consult for collaborative management.

Secondary Amenorrhea

Defined as the cessation of menstruation for the length of time three cycles would take, or for 6 months.

Laboratory tests

First test for beta human chorionic gonadotropin (hCG)

- If positive, the woman is pregnant
- If negative, obtain
  TSH
  Prolactin
  Progestational challenge (Provera 5 to 10 mg po qd for 5 to 10 days)

Normal TSH and prolactin levels coupled with a withdrawal bleed from the progestational challenge signals anovulation

If amenorrhea recurs, or if TSH or prolactin levels are elevated, or if woman has galactorrhea, consult for collaborative management or referral for endocrine evaluation

Notes

Vulvovaginal/Cervical Infections[5]*
General counseling for vulvovaginal/cervical infections

1. Etiology and course of infection
2. Use all medication as prescribed
3. Cotton underwear provides symptomatic relief
4. Loose clothing increases air circulation for symptomatic relief
5. Do not use tampons during treatment
6. Do not use feminine hygiene products, including douches
7. Use condoms or abstain from sexual intercourse during treatment
8. Use vaginal treatments at a time when you can remain lying down for several hours for best effect. Put a towel under your hips to avoid staining bedclothes; panty liners can be worn during the day

*Treatment regimens are according to the CDC *1998 Guidelines for Treatment of Sexually Transmitted Diseases.*

Candidiasis (Monilia)

Signs and symptoms
- Intense vulvovaginal itching
- Vulva often reddened, excoriated, edematous
- Discharge thick, white, cottage cheese–like; or thin and watery; or none
- White or white-yellow adherent plaques or patches on cervix or vaginal walls
- Generally no odor

Predisposing factors
- Pregnancy
- Broad-spectrum antibiotic therapy
- Hormone therapy, including contraceptives
- Immunosuppressant agents
- Diet high in refined sugars
- Diabetes

Unexplained recurrent infection warrants evaluation for HIV

Diagnosis
Clinical symptoms; vaginal pH $\leq$ 4.5; microscopic examination of potassium hydroxide (KOH) wet mount slide showing budding spores and pseudo-hyphae

Treatment
- Topically applied as intravaginal cream, vaginal tablets, or vaginal suppositories for 3–7 days depending on dosage
butoconazole (Femstat)
clotrimazole (Gyne-Lotrimin; Mylex-G)
miconazole (Monistat)
terconazole (Terazole-only by prescription)
- Oral medication
fluconazole (Diflucan) 150 mg po in a single dose (Category C; not for use in pregnancy per CDC)
- Self-care: plain yogurt douche or applicatorful bid × 7 days

Bacterial Vaginosis
Associated with preterm labor/preterm delivery and with postpartum endometritis

Signs and symptoms
- Discharge scanty or copious, thin, homogeneous, milky, gray or white in color
- Occasional vaginal irritation and pruritus and vulvar burning and pain
- Malodorous ("fishy")

Diagnosis
- Clinical symptoms
- Positive "whiff" test ("fishy" odor from amine release with KOH applied to specimen)

- Microscopic examination of wet mount slide shows clue cells, lack of lactobacilli, and very few white blood cells
- Elevated vaginal pH (>4.5)

Treatment (non-pregnant, in order of efficacy)
- Flagyl (metronidazole) 500 mg po bid x 7 days, or Clindamycin cream 2% 1 applicatorful intravaginal hs x 7 days, or
- metronidazole gel 0.75% 1 applicatorful intravaginal bid × 5 days or
- Flagyl (metronidazole) 2 g po in a single dose, or
- Clindamycin 300 mg po bid x 5 days

TREATMENT (PREGNANT)
- Flagyl (metronidazole) 250 mg po tid x 7 days, or alternatively
- Flagyl (metronidazole) 2 g po in a single dose, or
- Clindamycin 300 mg po bid x 7 days (Clindamycin cream is not recommended for use during pregnancy)

TREATMENT PRECAUTIONS
- Do not use alcohol when taking metronidazole or for 72 hours after completion of treatment
- Do not use latex or rubber products (condoms, diaphragm, cervical cap) for 72 hours after treatment with vaginal therapeutics

Sexually Transmitted Diseases[6]*
General counseling for sexually transmitted diseases:[||]

1. Etiology and course of infection
2. Potential effects on herself and baby (if pregnant) if not treated
3. Use all medication as prescribed
4. Partner(s) also must be treated

*Treatment regimens are according to the CDC *1998 Guidelines for Treatment of Sexually Transmitted Diseases.*
[||]See pp. 78–84 for a separate discussion of HIV and AIDS.

5. No sexual intercourse until both partners have completed therapy and are asymptomatic
6. Use of condoms/barriers after treatment

Trichomonal Vaginitis

- Primarily sexually transmitted
- Coexists with other sexually transmitted diseases—up to 50% of women with gonorrhea also have trichomonal vaginitis
- Evaluate for coexisting gonorrhea, chlamydia, and syphilis
- May be associated with PROM and PTL

Signs and symptoms

- Discharge is copious, may be frothy, thin or thick, and white, yellow-green, or gray
- Malodorous; may be "fishy"
- Vagina may be inflamed, ecchymotic, erythematous, excoriated
- Petechiae ("strawberry patches") on cervix or vaginal walls
- Dysuria
- Dyspareunia
- Postcoital bleeding
- Symptoms range from none to acute pelvic and lower abdominal pain with tender inguinal lymph nodes

Diagnosis

- Microscopic examination reveals motile trichomonads on wet mount slide
- May also be identified on Pap smear reports

Treatment

- Flagyl (metronidazole) 2 gm po × 1 dose or alternatively, 500 mg po bid × 7 days

Chlamydia

- Most prevalent STD in U.S.
- Often coexists with *Trichomonas* and *N. gonorrhoeae*

Signs and symptoms
- 50% of infected women are asymptomatic
- Mucopurulent cervical discharge
- Cervical edema or ectropion

Possible sequelae include
- Urogenital infections, which may be transmitted to the baby during the delivery and result in
  Opthalmia neonatorum
  Chlamydial neonatal pneumonia
- Infertility
- Ectopic pregnancy
- Premature rupture of the fetal membranes
- Preterm labor/preterm delivery

Diagnosis
  Positive cervical culture, ELISA, or gene probe

Treatment
(Treat presumptively for chlamydia in women being treated for gonorrhea)
- Azithromycin 1 g po × 1 dose (safety during pregnancy and lactation not established)
- Doxycycline 100 mg po bid × 7 days (contraindicated in pregnancy)
- Pregnancy Regimen:
  Erythromycin base 500 mg po qid × 7 days, or
  Amoxicillin 500 mg po tid × 7 days
- Erythromycin base erythromycin ethylsuccinate can be used during pregnancy; however, erythromycin estolate is contraindicated during pregnancy

Follow-up
  Test of cure not necessary with doxycycline or azithromycin unless reexposure is a risk. Otherwise repeat culture 3 weeks after completion of therapy.

Gonorrhea
- Routine culture is done for gonorrhea
- Often coexists with *Chlamydia trachomatis* and

Trichomonas
- Women with gonorrhea should also be screened for syphilis, because both have a high prevalence in the same risk populations

Signs and symptoms
- Generally asymptomatic when in lower genital tract
- In upper genital tract
  Acute PID
  Lower abdominal pain
  Urethritis
  Tenderness or purulent discharge from Bartholin's or Skene's glands or the urethra
  Yellow, mucopurulent, or purulent vaginal discharge
  History of unpleasant vaginal discharge, metrorrhagia, and menorrhagia

Possible sequelae
- Urogenital infections
- Infection of the eyes, oral mucosa, and joints (gonococcal arthritis)
- Infertility
- Premature rupture of the fetal membranes
- Preterm labor/preterm delivery
- Gonococcal ophthalmia neonatorum, which may cause blindness

Diagnosis
  Positive culture or gene probe

Treatment
- Ceftriaxone 125 mg IM in a single dose (1% lidocaine solution as a diluent may reduce pain of the injection)
- Spectinomycin 2 g IM in a single dose (for pregnant women who cannot tolerate ceftriaxone)
- Oral doses of cefixime (400 mg po × 1), ciprofloxacin (500 mg po × 1), or ofloxacin (400 mg

po × 1) may be used, but these agents are not bactericidally equivalent to ceftriaxone and may not be simultaneously effective against incubating syphilis; ciprofloxacin and ofloxacin are contraindicated for pregnant and lactating women and for persons under age 17

Follow-up
Test of cure not necessary (per the CDC).

Syphilis
- Routine screening is done for syphilis
- Pregnant women are screened at their first prenatal visit, at 28 weeks gestation, and at delivery.
- All women who have syphilis should be tested for HIV infection

Signs and symptoms

PRIMARY SYPHILIS
- Occurs 10 to 90 days after infection
- Begins as a painless papule that erodes to a highly infectious chancre (a chancre is a primary ulcerous lesion that is well demarcated, with induration of the base and circumference, and is filled with purulent discharge)
- Associated inguinal lymphadenopathy may exist

SECONDARY SYPHILIS
- Occurs 1 to 6 months after infection
- Papular rash on palms of hand and soles of feet, which may appear while lesion of primary syphilis is still present
- Patchy alopecia of head hair, eyebrows, and eyelashes
- Condylomata lata
- Mucous membrane lesions
- Symptoms of systemic illness, including low-grade fever, sore throat, hoarseness, malaise, headache, anorexia, and generalized adenopathy

LATENT SYPHILIS
- Early: occurs from time of infection to 1 year
- Late: occurs from 1 year after infection until onset of tertiary syphilis
- No clinical manifestations

TERTIARY SYPHILIS
- Occurs from 1 to 2 years after infection up to 30 or more years later
- Gumma: soft-tissue granuloma tumors in the liver, brain, heart, bone, and skin
- Cardiovascular: aortic valve disease, aortic aneurysm, coronary artery disease

NEUROSYPHILIS
- Occurs at any stage of syphilis
- Clinical symptoms of central nervous system (CNS) disease (e.g., cranial nerve palsies, personality changes, loss of reflexes)

Diagnosis
- Observation of *Treponema pallidum* spirochetes on darkfield examination
- Positive VDRL or RPR followed by positive FTA-ABS (antibody response is not measureable for 3 to 6 weeks after infection)
- A positive VDRL or RPR followed by a negative FTA-ABS may indicate a false-positive caused by an acute bacterial or viral infection (e.g., mononucleosis, leprosy, or malaria) or rheumatoid arthritis; repeat tests in 1 month
- VDRL or RPR nontreponemal serologic test results show a high titer or fourfold increase in titer when there is a new current infection; a low titer that does not increase when there is a previously treated infection; and a fourfold decrease in titer when there has been adequate treatment
- FTA-ABS treponemal test results may remain posi-

tive for life and should not be used to measure
stage of syphilis, degree of disease activity, or adequacy of treatment

Possible sequelae
- See signs and symptoms of tertiary syphilis
- Any stage of syphilis is transmitted through the
placenta to the fetus and, if untreated, results in a
40% rate of spontaneous abortion, stillbirth, or
perinatal death; another 40% give birth to babies
with congenital syphilis

Treatment
- Treatment is the same for pregnant and nonpreg-
nant women, and for those who are and are not
infected with HIV
- Treatment is in accord with the stage of syphilis
  PRIMARY, SECONDARY, AND EARLY LATENT SYPHILIS
- Benzathine penicillin G 2.4 million units IM in a
single dose; a second dose may be given 1 week
later if the woman is pregnant
- If a woman is allergic to penicillin and **not preg-
nant**
Doxycyclin 100 mg po bid × 14 days, or
Tetracycline 500 mg po qid × 14 days
  LATENT (LATE OR OF UNKNOWN DURATION)
  AND TERTIARY SYPHILIS
- Benzathine penicillin G 2.4 million units IM × 3
weekly doses (total of 7.2 million units)
- If a woman is allergic to penicillin and not preg-
nant
Doxycycline 100 mg po bid × 28 days
Tetracycline 500 mg po qid × 28 days

Follow-up
- Nonpregnant women: clinical and serologic evaluation at 6 and 12 (also 24 months if latent syphilis)
months after treatment

- Pregnant women: repeat serologic titers in third trimester and at delivery; notify anticipated pediatric health care provider
- Nonpregnant HIV-infected women: clinical and serologic evaluation at 3, 6, 9, 12 and 24 months after treatment
- Contact women's sexual partner(s) and treat presumptively if exposed within the preceding 90 days, even if partner is seronegative

Counseling specific to syphilis
- Signs and symptoms of progressive syphilis
- Signs and symptoms of Jarisch-Herxheimer reaction (acute febrile response to treatment with headache and myalgia for 12 to 24 hours)
- If pregnant: signs and symptoms of preterm labor; fetal movement counts; when to call the midwife

Genital Herpes Simplex Virus (HSV)
- Relatively common in women with HIV infection
- Monitoring for cervical cancer indicated

Signs and symptoms
- Primary episodes much more severe than recurrent episodes and last approximately 3 weeks
- Multiple single or clusters of thin-walled vesicles ulcerate, then crust and reepithelialize
- Ulcers, diffuse inflammation, and friability over the cervix, vaginal walls, perineum, labia, or anus
- Vaginal or urethral discharge
- Vulvar lesions extremely painful, may be accompanied by pruritus and severe edema
- Systemic symptoms: fever, malaise, headache and myalgia
- Very tender inguinal lymphadenopathy
- Recurrent episodes last about half as long with fewer vesicles, no systemic symptoms, and no inguinal lymphadenopathy

Diagnosis
History, clinical observation, and culture of exudate from lesion (80% sensitivity)

Possible sequelae
- Viral shedding and transmission of HSV from a mother with active infection to her newborn occurs during vaginal delivery in 50% of cases
- 60% of infected neonates (up to 28 days old) die
- Other neonates may have severe CNS or ocular damage

Treatment
- There is no cure for HSV
- Acyclovir (Zovirax) 400 mg po tid × 7–10 days may alleviate symptoms of a primary infection
- Acyclovir 400 mg tid × 5 days may relieve symptoms of an episodic recurrent infection
- Acyclovir 400 mg PO bid for up to 12 months may be used to suppress the frequency of recurrence, but should not be used by women who are or may become pregnant (not using contraceptives) during treatment

*Management of labor and delivery**
Most mothers of infants who acquire neonatal herpes lack histories of clinically evident genital herpes. The risk for transmission to the neonate from an infected mother appears highest among women with first episode genital herpes near the time of delivery, and is low (≤3%) among women with recurrent herpes who acquire genital HSV during the first half of pregnancy. The results of viral cultures during pregnancy do not predict viral shedding at the time of delivery, and such cultures are not routinely indicated.

At the onset of labor, all women should be carefully questioned about symptoms of genital herpes and should be examined. Women without symptoms or signs of genital herpes infection (or prodrome) may deliver their babies vaginally.

Infants delivered through an infected birth canal (proven by virus isolation or presumed by observation of lesions) should be followed carefully. Available data do not support the routine use of acyclovir as anticipatory treatment for asymptomatic infants delivered through an infected birth canal. Treatment should be reserved for infants who develop evidence of clinical disease and considered for those whose mothers acquired genital herpes near term.

All infants with evidence of neonatal herpes should be treated with systemic acyclovir. Acyclovir 30–60 mg/ kg/day for 10–21 days is the preferred regimen.

*Centers for Disease Control and Prevention. 1998 Sexually transmitted diseases treatment guidelines. MMWR 1998;47 (No. RR-1): 26.

Condylomata Acuminata (Genital Warts)
- Represents the clinical manifestation of HPV but is not an indication for colposcopy
- Women with condylomata acuminata should also be screened for syphilis, gonorrhea, chlamydia, trichomonas, and bacterial vaginosis

Signs and symptoms
- Vulvar, perineal, perianal, and vaginal warts are typically multiple, clustered, raised, and white with cauliflower appearance
- May have postcoital bleeding
- Cervical warts are usually single and flat
- A discharge is usually associated with the warts
- Condition is exaggerated by untreated vaginitis/ cervicitis
- Increase in size during pregnancy; regress after delivery

Diagnosis

Gross observation, history, and laboratory tests to rule out syphilitic condylomata lata

Treatment

- The goal of treatment is the removal of symptomatic warts
- High incidence of regrowth
- Treat any vaginal or cervical infection
- If topical treatments do not work, refer for possible cryotherapy or laser or surgical removal

Treatment (self-applied)

- Podofilox 0.5% solution or gel bid × 3 days followed by 4 days of no therapy; cycle repeated prn × 4 cycles. *Not for use in pregnancy*
- Imiquimod 5% cream 3 × a week up to 16 weeks. Wash treatment area with mild soap and water 6–10 hours after application. *Not for use in pregnancy*

Treatment (midwife-applied)

Podophyllin resin 10%–25% in compound tincture of benzoin. Allow to air dry. Wash off 1–4 hours after appplication to reduce local irritation. Protect surrounding tissue by covering with petroleum jelly before treatment. *Not for use in pregnancy or for anal, cervical, or oral warts.* Trichloroacetic acid (TCA) or bichloroacetic acid (BCA) 80%–90%. Allow to dry. May be used during pregnancy; use sodium bicarbonate or talc to counteract any burning.

Counseling specific for condylomata acuminata

- Careful cleaning to avoid trapping of discharge and feces and resulting foul odor; sitz bath after each bowel movement
- Frequent change of cotton underwear
- Importance of discussing warts with sexual partner(s); use condoms during sexual intercourse; no sexual intercourse during treatment

- Need for annual Pap smear
- Possible effect on delivery (cesarean section if extensive growth in vagina and over cervix; excessive bleeding if perineal warts are cut or torn)
- Possible effect on newborn and need to inform pediatric health care provider of diagnosis; baby has increased risk of developing laryngeal papillomatosis (vocal cord polyps)

Pelvic Inflammatory Disease (PID)

Usual causative organisms are *Neisseria gonorrhoeae, Chlamydia trachomatis,* or perhaps the organisms involved in bacterial vaginosis

Risk factors
- Exposure to causative organisms
- Multiple sexual partners
- Douching; IUD use
- Age 25 or younger

Use of condoms, or diaphragms and cervical caps with vaginal spermicides; decrease the risk of PID.

Signs and symptoms (may be subtle)
- Mild-to-severe lower abdominal pain
- Abnormal vaginal discharge
- Urethritis: dysuria, frequency, and urgency
- Metrorrhagia
- Peritonitis: fever; nausea and vomiting
- Cervical motion tenderness
- Bilateral adnexal tenderness and possible enlargement

Diagnosis
- Combination of presenting signs and symptoms with or without positive GC/chlamydia cultures
- Rule out other possible causes of lower abdominal pain
- Leukocytes outnumber epithelial cells on a wet mount

- Elevated erythrocyte sedimentation rate (ESR)

Possible sequelae
- Infertility
- Ectopic pregnancy
- Chronic lower abdominal pain
- If pregnant: preterm labor/delivery

Treatment
Must cover the likely pathogens plus anaerobic bacteria

INPATIENT TREATMENT
Physician consultation for intravenous broad-spectrum antimicrobial agents and possible laparoscopic evaluation is indicated when there is uncertain diagnosis, suspected pelvic abscess, severe symptoms, HIV, pregnancy, failed outpatient treatment, inability to comply with treatment and need for reevaluation within 72 hours, and for all adolescents

OUTPATIENT TREATMENT
- Ofloxacin 400 mg po bid × 14 days *plus* metronidazole 500 mg po bid × 14 days (this regimen is more expensive, but has broader coverage against anaerobic organisms than other regimens)
- If no clinical response in 72 hours, then hospitalize
- Sexual partner(s) should be treated empirically for both gonorrhea and chlamydia

Anaphylactic Shock
Signs and Symptoms
- Diffuse urticaria
- Rhinitis
- Laryngeal edema
- Dyspnea
- Wheezing
- Marked pallor

- Hypoxia
- Cyanosis
- Tachycardia
- Convulsions
- Hypotension
- Pupil dilatation
- Vascular collapse
- Cardiac arrest

Emergency Treatment

- Includes epinephrine, corticosteroids, and oxygen
- Intubation may be required
- Antihistamines are useful for lesser reactions or very early evidence from erythema or urticaria of a more severe reaction, which may lead to anaphylactic shock

Notes

HIV Infection and AIDS[7]

Routes of Transmission
- Sexual contact
- Mother to fetus or infant during pregnancy, birth, or breastfeeding
- Exposure to blood or body fluids

Risk Factors
- Multiple sexual partners
- Partner with multiple sex partners
- Intravenous drug use
- Partner using intravenous drugs
- Substance abuse
- Bisexual partner
- Transfusion with unscreened blood (before 1985 in U.S.)
- Occupation

Counseling and Testing
As a minimum, all women should be counseled and offered testing for HIV before and during pregnancy, at the initial gynecological exam when evaluated for STDs, and when their history indicates a need

Pretest counseling
- Routes of transmission
- Prevention
- Test interpretation
- Course of infection
- Resources
- Legal requirements

Posttest counseling of non-infected women
- Test results interpretation
- Assessment of risk factors
- Prevention of infection by safer behaviors
- Repeat testing as appropriate

Posttest counseling of infected women
- Test results interpretation

- Assessment of emotional and mental state
- Referral to care, including case management and medical care
- Issues of confidentiality and discrimination
- Prognosis
- Behavior changes to reduce transmission
- Protection from opportunistic infections

Laboratory tests

- HIV antibody tests are used to screen for infection
- Repeatedly positive EIA or ELISA assays are confirmed with Western blot before positive results are reported
- Both EIA and ELISA cross-react with other antibodies for a false-positive result
- Indeterminate Western blot tests should be repeated in 3 to 6 months
- False-positive Western blot results are rare
- Indeterminate results can also be confirmed by viral culture or PCR testing
- Both of these are sensitive, direct tests for virus presence but are expensive
- PCR measurement of viral load is also used in monitoring the course of infection and response to medication
- Viral culture, PCR, and p24 antigen assays are useful in obtaining early evidence of infant infection

Safety of sexual activities by category

LOW- OR NO-RISK ACTIVITIES

- Abstinence
- Self-masturbation
- Touching, hugging, massaging, caressing
- Social (dry) kissing

PROBABLY SAFE

- French (wet) kissing
- Mutual masturbation, if there are no lesions, sores, or cuts

- Vaginal sex with a male or female condom
- Fellatio with a condom
- Cunnilingus with a dental dam
- Anilingus with a dental dam
- Using one's own sex toys
- Anal sex with a condom and water-based lubricant
  PROBABLY UNSAFE
- Unprotected oral sex of any variety
  UNSAFE
- Vaginal intercourse
- Anal intercourse
- Anal intercourse with hand
- Sex with numerous partners

Use of condoms

- The use of condoms (male or female) or another adequate barrier has been demonstrated to significantly reduce the incidence of sexual transmission of HIV
- All women should be counseled to use a condom with all sexual activity until they are in a long-term, mutually monogamous relationship with an HIV-negative partner

  INSTRUCTIONS FOR CONDOM USE FOR HIV-POSITIVE WOMEN

1. Use a new condom every time you have sex, whether vaginal, anal, or oral.
2. Use only latex condoms.
3. Put the condom on as soon as the penis becomes erect, because HIV is present in pre-ejaculate fluid.
4. Remove the condom carefully immediately after ejaculation and discard it.
5. Use only water-based lubricants. Oil-based lubricants, such as baby oil, petroleum jelly, cold cream, or cooking oil, weaken the condom.
6. Avoid storing condoms where they might become overheated, such as in a back pocket or a hot car.

Condoms may weaken when exposed to prolonged extremes of temperature.

7. Use a condom even if both you and your partner have HIV infection, in order to avoid transmission of a different strain of HIV or another STD.

Care of Women with Early HIV Infection

In addition to the usual assessment of gynecological patients, the following should be emphasized

History
- Infections
- Fever
- Exposure to or symptoms of tuberculosis
- Substance abuse
- Sexual behaviors
- Changes in menses
- Weight loss
- Assessment of stability of social network
- Social service needs

Physical
- Temperature
- Fundoscopic evaluation
- Oral exam (for candidiasis)
- Lymph nodes
- Skin

Pelvic
- Pap smears at 6 months and then annually until symptomatic
- Pap smears every 6 months are required for history of HPV, SIL, or any cervical lesion
- Wet mounts at every exam
- Careful examination of the vulvar skin for VIN

Laboratory assessment of immune status
- CD4/CD8 absolute cell count and percentage every 6 months when above 600 CD4 cells/µl and every 3 months until 200 cells/µl

- Viral load testing with DNA or RNA PCR in coordination with primary care site
- PPD at initial assessment, with anergy panel; induration >5 mm is considered positive
- Whenever possible, tests should be coordinated with the woman's primary care site to decrease costs and spare the woman additional tests

Antiretroviral therapy

Currently, at least 10 medications are used singly and in a variety of combinations to treat HIV. Each has significant side effects; none has demonstrated effectiveness over a period of years, possibly due to the rate of viral mutation, as well as to intolerance of the adverse affects.

In pregnancy, consideration should be given to the woman's previous use of antiretrovirals, and her primary care provider consulted before discontinuing *any* medication, even in the first trimester. While the risks of these medications to the developing embryo are unknown, the risks to the mother of stopping may be severe. Anecdotal information regarding various regimens is available from the Antiretroviral Pregnancy Registry at 1-800-722-9292, ext. 38465.

Prophylaxis of opportunistic infections

- CD4 < 200: Bactrim 1 DS qd or qod, for PCP
- CD4 < 150: Rifabutin 300 mg po bid, for CMV retinitis

HIV infection: Pregnancy and the Infant

Pregnancy does not affect the course of HIV, nor does HIV affect the course of pregnancy, except in advanced disease. Early access to prenatal care, nutritional and social support, and availability of ZDV therapy for prevention of vertical transmission contribute to improved outcomes.

Counseling
- Reproductive choices

- Risks of transmission
- Availability of ZDV for self and infant
- Safer sex
- Low-intervention care to avoid theoretical risk associated with increased exposure to maternal blood and fluids
- Avoidance of breastfeeding
- Consideration of long-term planning

Additional laboratory tests during pregnancy (in collaboration with primary care provider)

- Screen for toxoplasmosis, CMV, HSV, rubella immunity, hepatitis, tuberculosis with PPD
- Obtain a CD4 and viral load at least every trimester
- Liver function tests (LFTs)
- When on ZDV, CBC every month

Use of zidovudine (Retrovir) to reduce perinatal transmission

Zidovudine (Retrovir) is also known as ZDV was formerly called AZT.

During pregnancy

Based on Protocol 076 for the AIDS Clinical Trial Group (ACTG), all women who are pregnant and HIV-positive should be offered ZDV after the first trimester.

Three regimens are often used

- ZDV 100 mg po 5 times a day (Protocol 076)
- ZDV 200 mg po tid

Women with anemia (Hgb less than 9) need to consider transfusion, erythropoetin, or stopping the medication.

In labor

ZDV is administered IV as a loading dose of 2 mg/kg of body weight over 1 hour, followed by 1 mg/kg of body weight per hour until delivery.

FOR THE NEWBORN

Oral ZDV syrup at 2mg/kg of body weight every 6 hours for 6 weeks, beginning within the first 12 hours of life.

SIDE EFFECTS OF ZDV

- Anemia
- Neutropenia
- Nausea
- Headaches
- Insomnia
- Rash
- Malaise

Screening tests for the newborn

- Culture and PCR ASAP after birth and at 1 and 4 months
- Two positive results are needed for confirmation of infection
- Negative results at 12 and 18 months confirm absence of infection
- The best results for infants of HIV-positive mothers are achieved when the pediatrician is knowledgeable about HIV

Signs and symptoms of pediatric HIV infection

- Early onset at 5 to 10 months
- Failure to thrive
- Diarrhea
- Otitis media
- Thrush
- Developmental delay
- Encephalopathy
- Opportunistic infections

Notes

Chapter 5

Preconception Care[1]

TABLE 5-1   *Preconception Care Assessment, Screening, and Education*

Assessment	Risk Screening	Education
Physical health	Chronic illnesses	Immunizations
	Infections	Fitness and
	STDs	exercise
	HIV	HIV counseling
	Dental work	
	needed	
	Labs, e.g., rubella	
	status, blood	
	type, hct	
Mental well-being	Psychological	Stress reduction
	problems	
	Family violence	
	Family/social	
	support	
Family planning	Infertility	Fertility/concep-
	Pregnancy losses	tion
		Timing pregnancy
		Discontinuing
		contraception

TABLE 5-1   Continued

Assessment	Risk Screening	Education*
Lifestyle	Substance abuse Socioeconomic risks Environmental hazards	Community resources
Nutrition	Eating disorders Obesity Underweight Pica Anemia	Diet for pregnancy Vitamin and mineral supplements Folic acid‖
Genetic history	Age Family history Exposure to teratogens Ethnic risk, e.g., Tay Sachs, Sickle cell	For specific problem
Occupation	Occupational hazards	For specific problem

*An essential component of preconception care is education for early and continuing prenatal care.

‖Preconception use of folic acid, 0.4 mg/day, reduces the risk of spina bifida and other neural tube defects.

Women with a personal or family history of any neural tube defect should consider taking 4.0 mg/day of folic acid beginning 4 weeks before planned conception through the first trimester.

Notes

Chapter 6

Antepartum

Initial Antepartal History[1]

Collect the woman's:

- Identifying information
- Past medical and primary care history
- Family history
- Menstrual history, including LMP for pregnancy dating
- Obstetric history
- Gynecologic history
- Sexual history
- Contraceptive history

Determine Gravida/Para

Gravida = number of times a woman has been pregnant

Para = number of pregnancies that terminated in birth of a fetus that reached the point of viability (28 weeks or 1000 grams)

First digit =   Number of term babies the woman has delivered (>36 weeks or >2500 gms)

Second digit =	Number of premature births (28 to 36 weeks or 1000 to 2499 gms)
Third digit =	Number of pregnancies ending in spontaneous or induced abortion prior to 28 weeks or <1000 gms
Fourth digit =	Number of children currently alive
Fifth digit =	Number of pregnancies that resulted in multiple births (rarely used)

Examples

Example 1: A Gravida 2 delivered a full-term baby with each pregnancy, both of whom are currently alive. She is a Para 2002.

Example 2: A Gravida 2 delivered a full-term baby who died at 6 months of age and aborted during her second pregnancy. She is a Para 1010.

Example 3: A Gravida 1 delivered premature twins, one of whom died. She is a Para 0201.

Example 4: A Gravida 6 delivered one full-term live birth, one full-term stillbirth, one premature live birth, and premature triplets, of whom two lived and one died, and she has had two abortions. She is a Para 2424. In this instance, it would be useful to use the fifth digit for the number of pregnancies that resulted in multiple births in order to clarify the first four numbers. With the five-digit system, she is a Para 24241.

In any of the above examples, if the woman were pregnant at the time of this summarizing of her obstetric history, her gravida number would increase by one to account for her present pregnancy.

Present Pregnancy History

1. Headaches
2. Dizziness
3. Visual disturbances

4. Syncope
5. Fever
6. Fatigue
7. Nausea
8. Vomiting
9. Heartburn
10. Breast changes
11. Leakage of colostrum
12. Shortness of breath
13. Abdominal pain
14. Back pain
15. Dyspareunia
16. Vaginal discharge
17. Vaginal bleeding
18. Dysuria
19. Urinary frequency
20. Constipation
21. Hemorrhoids
22. Leg cramps
23. Varicosities
24. Edema (ankle, pretibial, face, hands)
25. Infections (e.g., measles, flu, other viruses)
26. Drugs and medications
27. Roentgenography (exposure to x rays)
28. Accidents
29. Relationship status: support from significant other for pregnancy; presence or history of emotional, physical, or sexual abuse
30. Sexual satisfaction: sexual changes and the feelings of both partners toward any changes
31. Feelings about her pregnancy: effect on her life and her body image, feelings about the baby
32. Quickening (date of)
33. Any complaints, discomforts, or concerns other than those already discussed

A positive response to any of items 1 through 29 requires further exploratory history taking to ascertain the following:

1. When during the pregnancy this occurred; duration; recurrences
2. Specific location (if applicable)
3. Severity (if applicable)
4. Associated symptoms
5. Factors influencing the problem, either aggravating or relieving
6. Medical help (name of provider); diagnosis and treatment (if applicable)
7. Treatment or relief measures (self or medically initiated) and their effectiveness

Initial Antepartal Physical and Pelvic Examination[2]

A complete screening physical examination is done during the initial antepartal examination. In addition, the following is included in the abdominal examination of the pregnant woman:

1. Observation of any scars or bruises and inquiry to obtain explanation of them
2. Observation of linea nigra
3. Observation of abdominal striae
4. Determination of the lie, presentation, position, and variety of the fetus
5. Measurement of fundal height
6. Auscultation of fetal heart tones
7. Estimation of fetal weight
8. Observation or palpation of fetal movement

The only other additional information to be obtained from the physical examination is the woman's prepregnant weight and height at the time of her last menstrual period as well as her weight at the time of this examination.

A complete pelvic examination is done during the initial antepartal examination. This includes not only the speculum, bimanual, and rectovaginal examinations but also evaluation of the bony pelvis by clinical pelvimetry.

Pregnancy Tests[3]

Urine

These tests are available over the counter or from medical supply distributors.

A positive test is possible when there is a concentration of hCG in the urine of 25 mIUs, which has usually occurred by the time of missed menses, or 12 to 14 days after conception.

A positive test has a 99.5% predictive value for pregnancy. False-negatives can occur due to a low concentration of hCG, which may be caused by dilute urine, inaccurate dates, ectopic pregnancy, or a blighted ovum.

Serum beta-hCG

- Detected 7 to 11 days after conception
- Doubles every 2 days to about 10 weeks, then decreases
- Evaluation generally requires two values, 48 hours apart

Causes of low or falling hCG
  Spontaneous abortion
  Blighted ovum or missed abortion
  Viable pregnancy after 12 weeks
Causes of slow rising or leveling hCG
  Ectopic pregnancy
Causes of very rapid increase in hCG
  Multiple gestation
  Hydatidiform mole

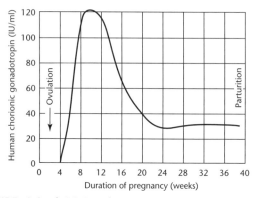

FIGURE 6-1   hCG Levels.

Diagnosis of Pregnancy[4]

History

1. Abrupt cessation of menstruation (presumptive)
2. Nausea and vomiting (presumptive)
3. Tingling, tenseness, nodularity, and enlargement of the breasts and enlargement of the nipples (presumptive)
4. Increased frequency of urination (presumptive)
5. Fatigue (presumptive)
6. Color changes of the breasts, i.e., darkening of the nipples and primary and secondary areolar changes (presumptive)
7. Appearance of Montgomery's tubercles or follicles (presumptive)
8. Continued elevation of the basal body temperature in the absence of an infection (presumptive)
9. Expression of colostrum from nipples (presumptive)
10. Excessive salivation (presumptive)
11. Chadwick's sign (presumptive)

12. Quickening (presumptive)
13. Skin pigmentation and conditions, e.g., chloasma, breast and abdominal striae, linea nigra, vascular spiders, palmar erythema (presumptive)

Physical Examination

1. Expression of colostrum from nipples (presumptive)
2. Color changes of the breasts (presumptive)
3. Nodularity, tenseness, and enlargement of the breasts and enlargement of the nipples (presumptive)
4. Appearance of Montgomery's tubercles or follicles (presumptive)
5. Enlargement of the abdomen (probable)
6. Palpation of the fetal outline (probable)
7. Ballottement (probable)
8. Fetal movement (positive or probable; authorities vary)
9. Fetal heart tones (positive)

Pelvic Examination

1. Enlargement of the uterus (probable)
2. Change in the shape of the uterus (probable)
3. Piskacek's sign (probable)
4. Hegar's sign (probable)
5. Goodell's sign (probable)
6. Palpation of Braxton Hicks contractions (probable)
7. Chadwick's sign (presumptive)

Laboratory Tests and Adjunctive Studies

1. Positive pregnancy test (probable)
2. Sonographic evidence of pregnancy (positive)

Dating the Pregnancy

There are three methods for dating a pregnancy:

1. "Sure" dates (the woman knows the date of the first day of her last normal menstrual period and has regular cycles)

2. Uterine sizing
3. Ultrasound

The determination of an estimated date of delivery (EDD) from two of these three methods must match to date the pregnancy with certainty.

Calculating the EDD from "Sure" Dates[5]

The EDD is calculated by *Naegele's rule,* in which 7 days are added to the date of the first day of the LMP and then 3 months are subtracted from that date. Naegele's rule is easiest to calculate by substituting numbers for months and days so that the first number stands for the month and the second number stands for the day. One must be careful to use the actual number of days in the month of the LMP when crossing over to another month. This is illustrated in the following example of calculating the EDD by Naegele's rule:

    5/28 (LMP of May 28)
  +   7 days
    6/4 (June 4—May has 31 days)
  −   3 months
  = 3/4 (March 4 of the next year, as 9 months have been added)

Uterine Sizing

A pregnancy between 6 and 16 weeks can be accurately dated within 1 to 2 weeks.

In a single pregnancy at 6 weeks

Shape: softening of the isthmus, slight globular shape

Size: handball or tangerine

In a single pregnancy at 8 to 10 weeks

Shape: overall globular shape with some uterine irregularity, particularly around one cornua (Piskacek's sign)

Size at 8 weeks: baseball or small orange
Size at 10 weeks: softball or large orange

In a single pregnancy at 12 weeks

Location: uterus at pelvic brim
Size: medium grapefruit

After 16 weeks, the size of the uterus is influenced by factors such as fetal growth and amniotic fluid volume. Other factors may affect the size and shape of the uterus early in pregnancy, such as multiple pregnancy, fibroids, missed abortion, hydatidiform mole, and multiparity.

TABLE 6-1   Accuracy of Dating by Ultrasound

Gestational Age (weeks)	Ultrasound Measurements	Range of Accuracy
<8	Sac size	±10 days
8–12	Crown rump length	±7 days
12–15	Crown rump length BPD	±14 days
15–20	BPD, HC, FL, AC	±10 days
20–28	BPD, HC, FL, AC	±2 weeks
>28	BPD, HC, FL, AC	±3 weeks

BPD = biparietal diameter

HC = head circumference

FL = femur length

AC = abdominal circumference

The Perinatal Collaborative Project and the National Institutes for Health (NIH) have recommended using a range of accuracy of ± 11 days prior to 20 weeks and ± 2 weeks at gestational ages greater than 20 weeks to take into consideration the variability in the accuracy of ultrasounds at different institutions.

Source: Used by permission of Eva Pressman MD, Johns Hopkins University School of Medicine.

Antepartal Revisit[6]

Chart Review

1. Name
2. Age
3. Parity
4. Weeks gestation by dates
5. Any significant finding from
   - Obstetrical history
   - Past medical and primary care history
   - Family history
   - Present pregnancy history
   - Initial physical examination
   - Initial pelvic examination
6. Any previously identified problems, treatment, and evaluation of the effectiveness of the treatment; review problem list
7. Any particular concerns and desires, plans made, and instructions provided
8. Specific medications, treatments, and dietary requirements for which the woman is presently responsible
9. Laboratory reports
   - Normality of results
   - Need to repeat any tests
   - Need for further investigation and tests

Interval History

1. Any concerns, complaints, questions, or problems
2. Headaches
3. Visual disturbances
4. Dizziness
5. Fever/chills
6. Nausea/vomiting
7. Fetal movement
8. Abdominal pain/contractions
9. Back pain
10. Dysuria

11. Vaginal discharge/leaking fluid
12. Vaginal bleeding
13. Constipation/hemorrhoids
14. Varicosities/leg ache
15. Leg cramps
16. Edema (ankle, pretibial, face, hands)
17. Exposure to any infectious diseases
18. Use of any medicines other than those prescribed (e.g., aspirin)
19. Any relationship changes, such as an increase in or initiation of abuse
20. Any medical care since last visit (e.g., doctor, emergency room); what for, diagnosis, treatment, continuing care

In addition, the woman is questioned about possible discomforts, concerns, and desire for information regarding the weeks gestation at the time of the revisit, as well as any plans she may have to attend classes on preparation for childbirth and parenthood (including breastfeeding).

Physical Examination

At each antepartal revisit, the following physical examination is done to detect any signs of complications and to evaluate fetal well-being.

1. Blood pressure (compare with baseline blood pressure obtained at the time of the initial visit; note blood pressure readings throughout pregnancy to date)
2. Weight (compare with prepregnant weight; note the number of pounds for the number of weeks since the last visit; note weight gain pattern)
3. Abdominal examination (see pp. 101–104)
4. CVA tenderness
5. Examination of the upper extremities for finger edema

6. Examination of the lower extremities for
   • Ankle and pretibial edema
   • Quadriceps (knee-jerk) deep tendon reflexes
   • Varicosities and Homan's sign, when indicated

Antepartal Laboratory Tests and Adjunctive Studies

Initial Visit

• Pap smear
• Gonorrhea culture
• Chlamydia culture
• Blood type (ABO)
• Rh factor
• Indirect Coombs' test/antibody titer
• Sickle cell prep or hemoglobin electrophoresis (found in an increasing number of settings)
• Tuberculin test (PPD), unless woman has a known previous positive test
• VDRL, RPR, or STS
• Hepatitis B surface antigen
• Rubella titer
• Varicella antibody screen
• Hemoglobin and hematocrit (some settings add CBC with differential, SMA 4, or SMA 12)
• Urinalysis for protein, glucose, and microscopic examination (some settings also order a culture)
• HIV testing (offered with counseling to all women)

15 to 18 Weeks

• Alpha-fetoprotein (AFP) triple screen (offered to all women, as close to 15 weeks as possible)

28 Weeks

• Diabetes screen
• Coombs' test/antibody titer (for Rh negative women if preceding titer was negative)

Third Trimester
- Hemoglobin and hematocrit
- VDRL

36 Weeks
- Gonorrhea culture
- Chlamydia culture
- Group B streptococcal screen (site-specific management plans may govern timing or population tested)

Obstetric Abdominal Examination[7]
1. Observation of any scars or bruises and inquiry to obtain explanation of them
2. Observation of linea nigra
3. Observation of abdominal striae
4. Determination of the lie, presentation, position, and variety of the fetus
5. Measurement of fundal height (see Table 6-2 and Figure 6-2)
6. Auscultation of fetal heart tones (see Figure 6-5)
7. Estimation of fetal weight
8. Observation or palpation of fetal movement

Abdominal palpation that includes the performance of Leopold's maneuvers (see Figures 6-3 and 6-4) is conducted for the following purposes.

1. Evaluation of uterine irritability, tone, tenderness, consistency, and any contractility
2. Evaluation of abdominal muscle tone
3. Detection of fetal movement
4. Estimation of fetal weight
5. Determination of fetal lie, presentation, position, and variety
6. Determination of whether the head is engaged

TABLE 6-2   Approximate Expected Fundal Height at Various Weeks of Gestation[8]

Weeks of Gestation	Approximate Expected Fundal Height
12	Level of the symphysis pubis
16	Halfway between symphysis pubis and umbilicus
20	1–2 fingerbreadths below umbilicus
24	1–2 fingerbreadths above umbilicus
28–30	One-third of the way between umbilicus and xyphoid process (three finger-breadths above umbilicus)
32	Two-thirds of the way between umbilicus and xyphoid process (three to four fingerbreadths below xyphoid process)
36–38	One fingerbreadth below xyphoid process
40	Two to three fingerbreadths below xyphoid process if lightening occurs

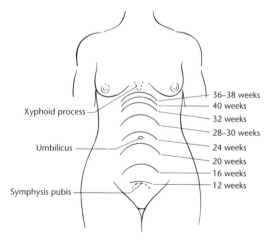

FIGURE 6-2   Approximate Normal Fundal Heights during Pregnancy.[8]

Leopold's Maneuvers

FIGURE 6-3
Palpation of Fetus in Left Occiput Anterior Position.

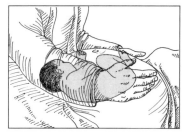

A. First maneuver.
Curve fingers of both hands around top of fundus. What is in the fundus?

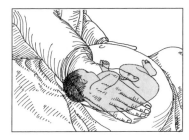

B. Second maneuver.
Place both hands on sides of uterus. Where are the baby's small parts?

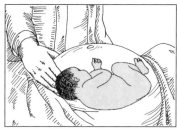

C. Third maneuver.
With thumb and middle finger of one hand press gently but deeply into the mother's abdomen immediately above the symphysis pubis and grasp the presenting part. What is the presenting part?

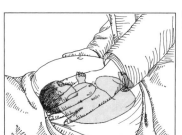

D. Fourth maneuver.
Place both hands on sides of lower uterus, press deeply and move fingertips towards pelvic inlet. Where is the cephalic prominence? Is the presenting part engaged?

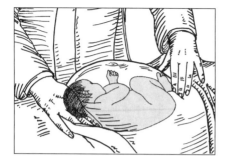

Combine Leopold's third maneuver with one hand and feel what is in the fundus with the other hand. Compare the two poles for final determination of lie and presentation.

FIGURE 6-4   Combined Pawlik's Grip.

Clinical Pelvimetry

Generally accepted findings from clinical evaluation of the bony pelvis that indicate pelvic adequacy include

> Forepelvis: rounded
> Sidewalls: straight
> Ischial spines: blunt
> Sacrospinous ligament: 2½ to 3 fingerbreadths
> Coccyx: movable
> Sacrum: hollow
> Diagonal conjugate: 11.5 cm or greater
> Pubic arch: 90° or greater (2 fingerbreadths)
> Intertuberous diameter: 8 cm or greater

Variations of the above findings in and of themselves would not indicate pelvic inadequacy. Remember these findings must be combined with other findings regarding inclination of the symphysis pubis, depth and angle of the sacrosciatic notch, alignment of the sacrum, and roominess of the posterior portion of the pelvis. The sum of all these findings gives a composite mental image of the total pelvis and its general type.

The individual pelvic architecture is then weighed against the estimated size of the fetus at term, the type of presenting part, and its position. A determination of pelvic adequacy is made from all these findings.

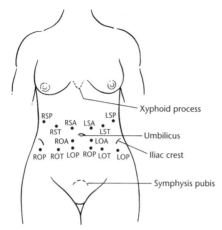

FIGURE 6-5 Location of the Point of Maximum Intensity of the Fetal Heart Tones for Specific Fetal Positions.[9]

Notes

Notes

Chapter 7

Fetal Assessment[1]

▣ Assessment for Structural and Genetic Abnormality

Maternal Serum Alpha-fetoprotein (MSAFP) and Triple Screen

Both MSAFP and triple screen are screening tests, not diagnostic tests. The triple screen (MSAFP, hCG, estradiol) offers improved identification of chromosomal anomalies over MSAFP alone. Offer MSAFP or triple screen to all women at 15 to 18 weeks menstrual age.

Normal values are based on

- Gestational age
- Maternal age
- Weight
- Race
- Diabetes, if present
- Multiple gestation

MSAFP is elevated when the fetus has an open neural tube defect and is decreased with Down Syndrome. See Figure 7-1 for management of abnormal MSAFP/triple screen test results.

Major Reasons for MSAFP Elevations*

- Underestimation of gestational age
- Multiple gestation
- Neural tube defects
- Ventral wall defects (omphalocele, gastroschisis)
- Renal anomalies (renal agenesis, urethral obstruction)
- Severe oligohydramnios
- Ectopic (including abdominal) pregnancy
- Fetal-maternal hemorrhage (may occur spontaneously or following CVS, amniocentesis or trauma)
- Underweight mother
- Black race
- Increased placental size

*Source: Reprinted with permission from R. L. Thomas and K. J. Blakemore. Evaluation of elevations in maternal serum alpha-fetoprotein: A review. *Obstet Gynecol Surv* 45(5):269–283, 1990.

Genetic Counseling

TABLE 7-1   Risk of Down Syndrome by Maternal Age *
80% of cases occur in mothers younger than 35 years.

Maternal Age	Risk
21	1/1667
23	1/1429
25	1/1250
27	1/1111
29	1/1000
31	1/909
33	1/625
35	1/385
37	1/227
39	1/137
41	1/82
43	1/50
45	1/30
47	1/18

*Source: Adapted with permission from S. G. Gabbe, J. Niebyl, and J. L.Simpson. *Obstetrics: Normal and Problem Pregnancies,* 3rd. ed. New York: Churchill Livingstone, 1996 p. 221.

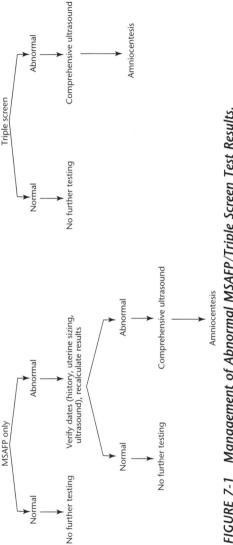

FIGURE 7-1 Management of Abnormal MSAFP/Triple Screen Test Results.
Most abnormal results are caused by inaccurate assessment of gestational age.

TABLE 7-2 Conditions Calling for Prenatal Diagnosis and Counseling*

Couples at an increased risk
   Maternal age >35 years
   Balanced chromosome rearrangement
   Previous child with chromosome abnormality
   Low MSAFP
Family history of birth defects and/or mental retardation
   Congenital heart disease
   Neural tube defect
   Cleft lip and/or palate
   Multiple congenital anomalies
   Mental retardation
Family history of known or suspected Mendelian genetic
   disorder
   Cystic fibrosis
   Hemophilia A
   Hemophilia B
   Duchenne muscular dystrophy
   Becker muscular dystrophy
Ethnicity
   African: Sickle cell disease; trait carriers
   Mediterranean/Indian: β-thalassemia
   Jewish: Tay-Sachs disease
Exposure to possible teratogens
   Alcohol
   Radiation
   Occupational chemical exposures
   Toxoplasmosis
   Rubella
   Cytomegalovirus
   Syphilis
Insulin-dependent diabetes mellitus
Epileptic disorder: drugs
Patients with low or high levels of MSAFP
Fetal abnormalities diagnosed by ultrasonogram
Consanguinity
Multiple pregnancy losses, stillbirth, infertility
Anxiety

*Source: P. Bauman and B. McFarlin. Prenatal diagnosis. *J Nurse-Midwifery* Elsevier Science Inc., 39(2, Supplement):37S. Copyright 1994 by the American College of Nurse-Midwives. Reprinted with permission.

▭ Fetal Assessment

Fetal Movement Counting (FMC)

All women may benefit from understanding that the fetus will develop its own behavioral pattern. If a woman notices a decrease or cessation in fetal movement, she should report this finding to the midwife. There are no specific "normal" numbers of fetal movements. A number of different time and number guidelines for fetal movement counting exist. Each clinician should choose and consistently use a single method.

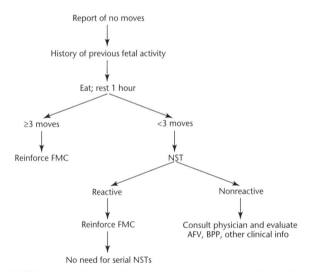

FIGURE 7-2   Fetal Movement Assessment Paradigm for Response to a Woman's Report of No or Decreased Fetal Movement.*

FMC, fetal movement counting; NST, nonstress test; AFV, amniotic fluid volume; BPP, biophysical profile.
*Source: By permission of Elsevier Science Inc. adapted from Antepartum fetal assessment: A nurse-midwifery perspective by C. L. Gegor, L. L. Paine, and T. R. B. Johnson. *J. Nurse-Midwifery* 36(3):157. Copyright 1991 by the American College of Nurse-Midwives. Reprinted with permission.

A Simple Method of FMC

1. Put 10 pennies in a cup.
2. Turn the pennies out on the table.
3. Put a penny back in the cup every time the baby moves.
4. If the pennies are not all back in the cup in 2 hours, call the midwife.

Daily FMC

Ask the woman to determine a time of day when the fetus is usually active and when she has time to focus on fetal movement. At the same time daily, determine how long it takes to identify 10 fetal movements.

If the time to reach 10 movements takes longer than usual or there are no movements, the woman should contact the midwife. FMC forms may be found in the accompanying textbook.[2]

Nonstress Test

Indications for the Nonstress Test (NST)[3]

Suspected IUGR in this pregnancy
History of IUGR in previous pregnancy
Pregestational diabetes
Gestational diabetes
Chronic hypertension
Pregnancy-induced hypertension
Preeclampsia
Multiple gestation
Oligohydramnios
Post dates
Rh isoimmunization
PROM
Decreased fetal movement
Previous stillbirth

Performance of the Nonstress Test (NST)[4]

- Place woman in a side-lying position (left or right side)

- Initiate external electronic fetal monitoring (both FHR and contraction monitoring)
- Identify the baseline FHR (minimum of 3 min)
- Continue monitoring for a minimum of 20 min

Note: A fetal event marker is not required for performance of the NST. FHR accelerations are associated with fetal movement, and maternal perception of this movement is not required.

Table 7-3   Interpretation Criteria for the Nonstress Test (NST)[5]

Interpretation	Criteria
Reactive	At least two accelerations of the FHR within a 20-min period that are off the baseline for at least 15 sec and that have a minimum amplitude of 15 bpm
Nonreactive	FHR tracing that fails to demonstrate adequate number or amplitude of FHR accelerations within any 20-min period
Inconclusive	A tracing of FHR that is uninterpretable because of difficulty obtaining the EFM tracing, or a tracing that does not demonstrate an FHR baseline (common with very vigorous fetuses)

Management of Results of Nonstress Test (NST)

- If the NST is reactive, the frequency of subsequent testing depends on the indication for testing.
- If the NST is nonreactive, further testing is indicated with a biophysical profile (BPP) or a contraction stress test (CST).
- If the NST is inconclusive, prolonging the NST until 45 minutes may clarify the tracing, or test further with a BPP.

Contraction Stress Test

Indications

Used as a follow-up to nonreassuring NST
High risk for IUGR
Post dates
Insulin-dependent diabetes
When ultrasound is not available for performance of BPP

Absolute Contraindications

Any time when labor is contraindicated
   Preterm labor
   Previous classical uterine incision
   Placenta previa

Procedures for Inducing Contractions for the Contraction Stress Test (CST)[6]

Breast stimulation

Stimulation of one nipple, through the clothing
2 minutes' stimulation
5 minutes' resting
Do not stimulate through a contraction
If not successful within 45 min, perform OCT

Oxytocin challenge test (OCT)

Intravenous infusion, D5/0.2NS keep-vein-open rate
Oxytocin solution: 1 mIU/min pitocin in 500 cc D5/0.2NS per infusion pump
Titrate beginning at 1 mIU/min
Increase 1 mIU/min every 15 min
Continue until adequate contraction pattern or abnormal FHR patterns

Contraction Stress Test Interpretation Criteria[7]

Before interpreting of FHR patterns, the EFM strip must demonstrate 3 contractions within 10 min with a minimum of 40 sec off the baseline. (It is unnecessary for the woman to perceive the contractions.)

Interpretation

Negative (reassuring): FHR stable, without evidence of late decelerations

Positive (nonreassuring): Repetitive late decelerations following each contraction

Equivocal: Unable to obtain satisfactory tracing

Uterine hyperstimulation

Nonrepetitive decelerations

Management of Result of CST

- If the CST is negative (reassuring), another CST is not necessary for 7 days.
- If the CST is positive (nonreassuring), the results need to be interpreted within the context of the woman's overall clinical picture, because there is a 30% false-positive rate. This assessment will determine whether to follow-up with a BPP, or to repeat a CST within 24 hours, or to take immediate steps to deliver the baby.
- If the CST is equivocal with results confounded by hyperstimulation or nonrepetitive decelerations, the CST should be repeated within 24 hours or a BPP should be done immediately. If the BPP results are reassuring, the CST need not be repeated.

Notes

TABLE 7-4 Indications for BPP and Suggested Testing Frequency

Diagnosis	Frequency of BPP/NST	Begin at Gestational Age (weeks)
IUGR or suspected uteroplacental insufficiency	Weekly/twice weekly	28
Diabetes, insulin dependent	Weekly/twice weekly	28
Diabetes, gestational, diet only	Weekly	36
Hypertension, chronic	Weekly	34–36
Hypertension, uncontrolled, PIH	Weekly/twice weekly	28
Twins, normal growth	Weekly	34–36
Twins, discordant growth	Weekly/twice weekly	28
PROM	Twice weekly or daily	Onset of PROM
Previous loss	Weekly	34 (or 2 wks earlier than previous loss occurred)
Postdates ≥41 weeks	Twice weekly	40–41

TABLE 7-5 **BPP Criteria (Modified Manning)***
Maximum time: 30 minutes

Biophysical Category	Criteria Present (score 2 points)	Criteria Absent (score 0 points)
Fetal tone	At least one episode of extension with return to flexion of fetal limbs or spine, clenched fist, sucking, and swallowing	No evidence of tone, open hands, outstretched limbs
Fetal movement	At least 3 episodes of extension and flexion of fetal limbs or full body rolling	2 or fewer episodes of movement
Fetal breathing movements	At least 30 seconds of continuous respiratory activity	No breathing or less than 30 seconds of respiratory activity
Fetal heart rate reactivity	Reactive NST (2 accelerations in 20 min of 15 sec duration × 15 bpm amplitude)	Nonreactive NST
Amniotic fluid volume	At least one single pocket 2 cm or more depth, or AFI >5.0 cm	Oligohydramnios

**Source:* Adapted from C. L. Gegor. Third trimester ultrasound for nurse-midwives. *J Nurse-Midwifery,* 38(2):29–41. Copyright American College of Nurse-Midwives. Reprinted with permission.

TABLE 7-6 Obstetrical Management Based on Modified Manning BPP Results*

BPP Score	Assessment	PMR|| in 1 Week	Management
10/10 or 8/10, normal AFV	Low risk for perinatal asphyxia	<1/1000	Repeat BPP in one week. (If fetus at high risk for UPI, twice weekly NST may be indicated. If postdates, twice weekly BPP may be indicated.)
8/10, abnormal AFV	High risk for perinatal asphyxia	89/1000	Consider delivery for fetal indications. May consider maternal hydration and reevaluate AFV within 24 hr.
6/10, normal AFV	Equivocal results	Variable	If fetus is mature, consider delivery for fetal indications. If fetus is immature, repeat BPP within 24 hr.
6/10, abnormal AFV	High risk for perinatal asphyxia (if membranes are intact and fetus is known to have functioning kidneys)	89/1000	If fetus is mature, deliver for fetal indication. If fetus is immature, maintain constant observation, repeat

			BPP within 24 hr. Consult or refer for medical management.
4/10	High risk for perinatal asphyxia	91/1000	Delivery recommended for fetal indications. Consult or refer for medical management.
2/10	Perinatal asphyxia almost certain	125/1000	Delivery recommended for fetal indications. Consult or refer for medical management.
0/10	Perinatal asphyxia certain	600/1000	Delivery recommended for fetal indications. Consult or refer for medical management.

Source: Reprinted by permission from F. A. Manning, and C. R. Harmon. The fetal biophysical profile. In R. D. Eden and F. H. Boehm. *Assessment and Care of the Fetus: Physiological, Clinical, and Medicolegal Principles.* Norwalk, CT: Appleton and Lange, 1990. Chapter 28, Table 28-2, p. 390.
‖Perinatal mortality

Modified Biophysical Profile (NST and AFI)

When the NST is reactive (2)

Reactivity means the fetus is moving (2), and if moving, there is fetal tone (2).

Therefore, the reactive NST is equivalent to a **BPP score of 6.**

Amniotic fluid index (AFI) of >5.0 cm = **BPP score of 2**

The predictive value of a modified BPP when the NST is reactive and the AFI is >5.0 cm is equivalent to a full BPP score of 8/10.

If the NST is nonreactive or the AFI is <5.0 cm, a full BPP must be done.

Amniotic Fluid Volume (AFV)

Risk factors for oligohydramnios

- PROM
- IUGR
- Postdates
- Fetal anomaly (esp., renal agenesis, polycystic kidneys, obstructive uropathy)
- Maternal systemic illness
- Insulin-dependent diabetes
- Maternal hydration

Single pocket method (measured in vertical dimension)

- Normal: 2.0 cm of fluid or more
- Oligohydramnios: no single pocket of fluid of at least 2.0 cm

Amniotic fluid index (AFI)

The AFI is a semiquantitative method of assessing quantity of amniotic fluid.

Procedure for Performing an AFI[8]

Place woman in supine position

Identify four quadrants of maternal abdomen

Scan with the transducer placed perpendicular to the floor, aligned longitudinally with the maternal spine

Measure vertical depth of largest clear pocket of amniotic fluid

AFI = sum of four quadrants

Normal values for AFI
"Rule of thumb" at term
   <5.0 cm = oligohydramnios
   >23 cm = polyhydramnios

TABLE 7-7   Amniotic Fluid Index for Normal Pregnancy by Gestational Age*

Gestational Age (wks)	Low Normal (cm)	High Normal (cm)
28	8.6	24.9
29	8.4	25.4
30	8.2	25.8
31	7.9	26.3
32	7.7	26.9
33	7.4	27.4
34	7.2	27.8
35	7.0	27.9
36	6.8	27.9
37	6.6	27.5
38	6.5	26.9
39	6.4	25.5
40	6.3	24.0
41	6.3	21.6
42	6.3	19.2

*Source: Adapted by permission from T. R. Moore and J. E. Cayle. The amniotic fluid index in normal human pregnancy. *Am J Obstet Gynecol* 1990; 162:1168–73.

Obstetrical Ultrasound

Indications for Obstetrical Ultrasound*

Estimated gestational age for patients with uncertain clinical dates

Evaluation of fetal growth

Vaginal bleeding of undetermined etiology

Determination of fetal presentation

Suspected multiple gestation

Adjunct to amniocentesis

Significant uterine size/clinical dates discrepancy

Pelvic mass

Suspected hydatidiform mole

Suspected ectopic pregnancy

Adjunct to special procedures, e.g., fetoscopy, cordocentesis, chorionic villus sampling, in vitro fertilization, cervical cerclage placement

Suspected fetal death

Suspected uterine abnormality

Localization of intrauterine contraceptive device

Surveillance of ovarian follicle development

Biophysical evaluation for fetal well-being

Observation of intrapartum events, e.g., version/extraction of second twin

Manual removal of placenta

Suspected polyhydramnios or oligohydramnios

Suspected abruptio placenta

Adjunct to external cephalic version

Estimation of fetal weight

Abnormal serum alpha-fetoprotein value

Follow-up observation of identified fetal anomaly

Follow-up evaluation of placenta location for identified placenta previa

History of previous congenital anomaly

Serial evaluation of fetal growth in multiple gestation

Evaluation of fetal condition in late registrants for prenatal care

*Source: National Institutes of Health, 1984.

Components of a Basic Obstetrical Ultrasound Examination*

First-trimester sonography

Scanning may be performed abdominally or vaginally
The following assessments should be made

Gestational sac location

Identification of embryo

Crown-rump length

Presence or absence of fetal cardiac activity

Fetal number

Evaluation of the uterus and adnexal structures

Second- and third-trimester sonography

Unless technically impossible, the following aspects should be assessed during a basic ultrasound examination

Fetal number

Fetal presentation

Documentation of fetal cardiac activity

Placental localization

Amniotic fluid volume assessment

Gestational dating, using at least two fetal parameters

Detection and evaluation of maternal pelvic masses

Survey of fetal anatomy for gross malformations

Source: Adapted by permission from American College of Obstetricians and Gynecologists. *Ultrasonography in Pregnancy.* Technical Bulletin No. 187. Washington, DC, © ACOG, December 1993.

Indications for Limited Scans*

A limited ultrasound examination may be appropriate and desirable in certain circumstances, such as when specific information is required or the clinical situation is urgent. A limited examination may be useful for the following tasks

Assessment of amniotic fluid volume

Conducting fetal biophysical profile

Conducting ultrasonography-guided amniocentesis

Determination of external cephalic version
Confirmation of fetal life or death
Localization of placenta in antepartum hemorrhage
Confirmation of fetal presentation

Source: Adapted by permission from American College of Obstetricians and Gynecologists. *Ultrasonography in Pregnancy.* Technical Bulletin No. 187. Washington, DC, © ACOG, December 1993.

*Minimum Components of Limited Obstetrical Ultrasound, Second and Third Trimester**

Fetal number
Fetal cardiac activity
Fetal lie
Placental location
Biophysical profile parameters
Amniotic fluid volume

Source: Reprinted by permission from American College of Nurse-Midwives. *Limited Obstetrical Ultrasound in the Third Trimester.* Clinical Bulletin No. 1. Washington, DC, ACNM, 1996.

Notes

Chapter 8

Nutrition in Pregnancy[1]

▬ Weight Gain

Body Mass Index (BMI)

The Institute of Medicine's Subcommittee on Nutritional Status and Weight Gain During Pregnancy proposed that gestational weight gain be predicated on a woman's prepregnancy body mass index (BMI, or "weight for height"; see Table 8-1).

The method for determining optimum weight gain during pregnancy is first to ascertain the woman's prepregnancy BMI. The recommended range of total weight gain during pregnancy is determined by the prepregnancy BMI. The woman should achieve at least the lower limit of the weight gain specified by her BMI. The total weight gain for twin pregnancies consistent with good outcomes is 35 to 45 lbs. The recommended weekly weight gain in the second and third trimesters is 1.5 lb/wk. Caloric intake is determined by multiplying the woman's optimal nonpregnant body weight in kilograms by 35 kcal and then adding 300 kcal to the total.

125

TABLE 8-1   Abbreviated Body Mass Index (BMI)*

Height (ft, in)

Weight (lb)	4'10"	5'0"	5'2"	5'4"	5'6"	5'8"	5'10"	6'0"	6'2"
125	26	24	23	22	20	19	18	17	16
130	27	25	24	22	21	20	19	18	17
135	28	26	25	23	22	21	19	18	17
140	29	27	26	24	23	21	20	19	18
145	30	28	27	25	23	22	21	20	19
150	31	29	27	26	24	23	22	20	19
155	32	30	28	27	25	24	22	21	20
160	34	31	29	28	26	24	23	22	21
165	35	32	30	28	27	25	24	22	21
170	36	33	31	29	28	26	24	23	22
175	37	34	32	30	28	27	25	24	23
180	38	35	33	31	29	27	26	25	23
185	39	36	34	32	30	28	27	25	24
190	40	37	35	33	31	29	27	26	24
195	41	38	36	34	32	30	28	27	25
200	42	39	37	34	32	30	29	27	26
205	43	40	38	35	33	31	29	28	26
210	44	41	38	36	34	32	30	29	27
215	45	42	39	37	35	33	31	29	28
220	46	43	40	38	36	34	32	30	28
225	47	44	41	39	36	34	32	31	29
230	48	45	42	40	37	35	33	31	30

*BMI is defined as body weight (in kg) divided by height (in m²).

The intersection of the woman's weight (row) and height (column) is her BMI.

Source: Adapted from Wyeth-Ayerst Laboratories, 1996. Courtesy of Wyeth-Ayers Laboratories, Philadelphia, PA.

TABLE 8-2   Recommended Total Weight Gain Ranges for Pregnant Women by Prepregnancy BMI*

BMI Category	Weight Gain	
	kg	*lb*
Low (BMI <19.8)	12.5–18	28–40
Normal (BMI of 19.8 to 26.0)	11.5–16	25–35
High (BMI >26.0 to 29.0)‖	7.0–11.5	15–25

*Young adolescents and black women should strive for gains at the upper end of the recommended range. Short women (<157 cm, or 62 in.) should strive for gains at the lower end of the range.
‖The recommended target weight gain for obese women (BMI >29.0) is at least 6.0 kg (15 lb).
**Source:* Adapted with permission from *Nutrition During Pregnancy.* Copyright 1990 by the National Academy of Sciences. Courtesy of National Academy Press, Washington, DC.

Higgins Intervention Methodology

To determine normal weight requirements for a mother 20 years of age or more, the client's height and body frame are located on Table 8.3 and the ideal weight is ascertained on the basis of these data.

The client's ideal weight and her activity level are now located on the 1948 Canadian Dietary Standard (Table 8-4), and the woman's nonpregnant calorie and protein requirements are ascertained.

After 20 weeks' gestation, 500 calories and 25 g of protein are added to the woman's daily nonpregnant calorie and protein requirements, as determined above. These now become her normal pregnancy calorie and protein requirements.

If the pregnancy is a multiple gestation, 500 calories and 25 g of protein are added for each fetus.

TABLE 8-3   Desirable Weights for Women*

Height	Small Frame (lbs, range and average)	Medium Frame (lbs, range and average)	Large Frame (lbs, range and average)
4'10"	92–98 (95)	96–107 (101.5)	104–119 (111.5)
4'11"	94–101 (97.5)	98–110 (104)	106–122 (114)
5'0"	96–104 (100)	101–113 (107)	109–125 (117)
5'1"	99–107 (103)	104–116 (110)	112–128 (120)
5'2"	102–110 (106)	107–119 (113)	115–131 (123)
5'3"	105–113 (109)	110–122 (116)	118–134 (126)
5'4"	108–116 (112)	113–126 (119.5)	121–138 (129.5)
5'5"	111–119 (115)	116–130 (123)	125–142 (133.5)
5'6"	114–123 (118.5)	120–135 (127.5)	129–146 (137.5)
5'7"	118–127 (122.5)	124–139 (131.5)	133–150 (141.5)
5'8"	122–131 (126.5)	128–143 (135.5)	137–154 (145.5)
5'9"	126–135 (130.5)	132–147 (139.5)	141–158 (149.5)
5'10"	130–140 (135)	136–151 (143.5)	145–163 (154)
5'11"	134–144 (139)	140–155 (147.5)	149–168 (158.5)
6'0"	138–148 (143)	144–159 (155.5)	153–173 (163)

*In using this table, be sure to use the height figure 2 inches taller than your client measures in her stocking feet, since the heights in the table include shoes with 2-in. heels.

Source: 1959 Actuarial Tables. Courtesy of the Metropolitan Life Insurance Company.

TABLE 8-4 Canadian Dietary Standard for Female Adults, 1948

Ideal Body Weight (lb)	Sedentary Activities		Moderate Activities		Heavy Activities	
	Calories	Protein (g)	Calories	Protein (g)	Calories	Protein (g)
80	1600	40	1900	40	2400	40
85	1650	43	1950	43	2450	43
90	1700	45	2000	45	2500	45
95	1750	48	2050	48	2550	48
100	1800	50	2100	50	2600	50
105	1875	51	2175	51	2675	51
110	1950	53	2250	53	2750	53
115	2025	54	2325	54	2825	54
120	2100	55	2400	55	2900	55
125	2150	57	2450	57	2950	57
130	2200	58	2500	58	3000	58
135	2250	59	2550	59	3050	59
140	2300	60	2600	60	3100	60
145	2350	63	2650	63	3150	63
150	2400	65	2700	65	3200	65
155	2450	68	2750	68	3250	68
160	2500	70	2800	70	3300	70

To determine normal weight requirements for a mother 19 years of age or less, the client's age is located on the 1958 U.S. Recommended Daily Allowance (RDA) calorie and protein requirements for women under age 19. This determines the woman's nonpregnant calorie and protein requirements.

TABLE 8-5   Calorie   and   Protein   Requirements   for   Women under 19, U.S. RDA, 1958

Age (yr)	Calories	Protein (g)
13–15	2600	80
16–19	2400	75

Source: From the Food and Nutrition Board, National Academy of Sciences—National Research Council, 1958.

Determination of Additional Corrective Allowances
Additional corrective allowances of calories and protein are given for three categories of identifiable nutritional conditions that may adversely affect pregnancy outcome if not considered

1. Undernutrition
2. Underweight
3. Nutritional stress

Each requires a separate addition to the daily normal pregnancy requirements for protein and calories.

Undernutrition assessment and corrective allowance
Undernutrition is defined as a deficit in protein between the normal pregnancy protein requirements for an individual woman and her actual dietary intake of protein, as determined by calculations performed on the data collected from a diet history. The corrective allowance is as follows

Protein—the number of grams of protein deficit is added to the daily normal pregnancy requirements for protein

Calories—for each gram of protein deficit, 10 calories are added to the daily normal pregnancy requirements for calories (i.e., 10 calories × the number of grams of protein deficit = the total calorie addition)

Underweight assessment and corrective allowance

Underweight is defined as the mother's prepregnant weight being 5% or more under the ideal weight as determined from the table of desirable weights. The corrective allowance is as follows

Protein—20 g per day
Calories—500 calories per day

Both the protein and calorie corrections are added to the daily normal pregnancy requirements for protein and calories. This corrective allowance of protein and calories will permit an additional weight gain of 1 lb per week and should be continued for the number of weeks equivalent to the number of pounds the mother was underweight before conception. The allowance may be cut in half if needed for a weight gain of ½ lb per week or increased to a maximum addition of 1000 calories and 40 g protein daily if a weight gain of 2 lb per week is needed in order to make up the deficit by the time of delivery.

*Nutritional stress assessment
and corrective allowance*

Nutritional stress is defined as the existence of one or more of the following conditions

Pernicious vomiting
Pregnancy spacing less than 1 year apart
Poor obstetrical history

Failure to gain 10 lb by the twentieth week of gestation

Serious emotional upset or problems

The corrective allowance is an additional 200 calories and 20 g protein for each stress condition present (up to a maximum allowance of 400 calories and 40 g protein) to be added to the daily normal pregnancy requirements for protein and calories.

TABLE 8-6   *Summary Format for Calculating Calorie and Protein Requirements During Pregnancy[2]*

Category	Calories	Protein (g)
Nonpregnant requirements	————	————
Addition for pregnancy (after 20th week)	500	25
Undernutrition corrective allowance	————	————
Underweight corrective allowance	————	————
Nutritional stress corrective allowance	————	————
Total	————	————

▭ Nutritional Needs in Pregnancy

Nutritional High-Risk Populations
Women who:

- Use tobacco
- Use alcohol
- Use caffeine or coffee
- Use marijuana
- Use cocaine or any other illicit substances
- Have lactose intolerance
- Have multiple gestations
- Are strict vegetarians

Iron Supplementation

- If required in pregnancy, 30 mg elemental iron (150 mg ferrous sulfate, 300 mg ferrous gluconate, or 100 mg ferrous fumarate) daily
- Nonheme iron comprises the majority of dietary iron
- Meat and ascorbic acid–rich foods enhance absorption of nonheme iron
- Tea, coffee, and milk reduce absorption of nonheme iron
- Iron is best taken between meals with orange juice

Dietary Sources of Major Nutrients

TABLE 8-7   Iron

RDA: Pregnancy, 30 mg; breastfeeding, 15 mg

Food	Quantity	Iron (mg)
Clams	3 oz	24
Pork liver	3 oz	15
Oysters	3 oz	11
Soybeans	1 c*	9
Tofu	4 oz**	7–13
Beef liver	3 oz	6
Mussels	3 oz	6
Molasses, blackstrap	2 Tbs	6
Almonds	2/3 c	5
Chickpeas	1 c*	5
Roast beef	3 oz	4
Beans, white	8 oz*	4
Prunes, dried	6 oz	4
Prune juice	8 oz	3
Spinach	1 c*	3
Raisins	1/2 c	3
Veal, broiled/baked	3 oz	3

*Cooked
**Firm type

Folic Acid Supplementation

- 0.4 mg to 0.8 mg/day
- Reduces megaloblastic anemia
- Use with iron if woman is anemic
- Reduces risk of neural tube defects if taken before conception and during first 6 wks of pregnancy

Vitamin C Supplementation

- 250 mg/day taken with meals
- Enhances absorption of nonheme iron
- May enhance absorption of iron supplements
- May be prophylactic for postpartal hemorrhage

TABLE 8-8   Vitamin C

RDA: Pregnancy, 70 mg; breastfeeding, 95 mg

Food	Quantity	Vitamin C (mg)
Guava	1 lg	242
Green pepper	1 lg	128
Kale, cooked	1 cup	93
Broccoli, cooked	2/3 c	90
Collard greens, cooked	1/2 c	76
Strawberries	2/3 c	59
Papaya	1/2 c	56
Lemon	1 med	53
Orange	1 sm	50
Spinach, raw	3 1/2 oz	51
canned	1/2 c	28
Grapefruit	1/2 med	38
Tangerine	1 med	31
Sweet potato	1 sm	22
Tomato	1 sm*	23
Tomato, canned	1/2 c	20
Potato, white baked w/skin	1 med	20
Tomato juice	1/2 c	16

*Raw

TABLE 8-9 Calcium
RDA: 1200 mg during pregnancy and breastfeeding

Food	Quantity	Calcium (mg)
Ricotta	1 c	669
Carnation Instant Breakfast with 1% milk	8 oz	500
Sardines	3½ oz	437
Yogurt, low fat plain	1 c	415
Yogurt, low fat fruit varieties	1 c	350
Collard greens	1 c	357
Cooked rhubarb	1 c	348
Lowfat 1% milk	8 oz	300
Tums E-X	1 tab	300
Whole milk	8 oz	288
Buttermilk	8 oz	285
Chocolate 2% milk	8 oz	284
Spinach, cooked	1 c	278
Molasses, blackstrap	2 Tbsp	274
Firm tofu made with calcium sulfate	4 oz	250–265
Swiss cheese	1 oz	272
Provolone	1 oz	214
Cheddar cheese	1 oz	204
Mozzarella	1 oz	185
Sesame seeds	2 Tbsp	176
Ice cream, vanilla, 16% fat	1 c	151
Salmon, canned with bones	3 oz	133
Peanuts, oil roasted	1 c	126
American cheese	1 oz	124
Regular tofu, made with calcium sulfate	4 oz	120–392
Tahini (sesame paste)	1 oz	119
Sherbet	1 c	103
Tofu made with nijare	4 oz	80–146
Cottage cheese	4 oz	70
Hummus	½ c	62
Almonds, blanched	1 oz	50
Chickpeas	½ c	40
Broccoli	½ c	36

TABLE 8-10   Folic Acid

RDA: 400 mcg before and during pregnancy

Food	Quantity	Folic Aid (mcg)
Meats		
Liver	3½ oz	220
Egg	1	22
Ground beef	3 oz	8
Turkey	3 oz	6
Chicken	3 oz	5
Ham	3 oz	5
Fish and shellfish		
Oysters, raw	1 c	25
Crabmeat	1 c	21
Scallops	6	15
Haddock	3 oz	14
Salmon	3½ oz	14
Cod	3½ oz	10
Shrimp	3½ oz	5
Fruit and fruit juices		
Orange juice	8 oz	100
Grapefruit juice	8 oz	52
Cantaloupe	1 c	48
Orange	1 med	45
Strawberries	1 c	26
Banana	1 med	22
Pineapple, fresh	1 c	16
Grapefruit	½ med	15
Pear	1 med	12
Vegetables		
Asparagus	½ c	108
Romaine lettuce	1 c	76
Broccoli	½ c	65
Spinach	½ c	54
Peas	½ c	51
Brussels sprouts	½ c	47
Tomatoes, canned	1 c	35
Iceberg lettuce	1 c	31
Baked potato	1 med	22

(Continued)

TABLE 8-10   (Continued)

Food	Quantity	Folic Aid (mcg)
Legumes		
Navy beans	1 c	255
Chickpeas, canned	1 c	160
Kidney beans, canned	1 c	126
Baked beans	1 c	61
Nuts		
Almonds	1 oz	88
Peanuts	1 oz	24
Cashews	1 oz	20
Walnuts	1 oz	19
Pistachios	1 oz	17
Pecans	1 oz	12
Bread and grain products		
Oatmeal, instant and fortified	¾ c	150
Wheat germ	¼ c	100
Bran muffin	1	19
Whole wheat bread	1 slice	16
Macaroni	1 c	10
White bread	1 slice	10
Rice, brown or white	1 c	8
Milk and milk products		
Cottage cheese	1 c	28
Yogurt	1 c	25
Milk	1 c	13
Cheddar cheese	1 oz	5
Ice cream	1 c	3
American cheese	1 oz	2
Other		
Brewer's yeast	1 Tbsp	313
Cereals		

Many cereals are fortified with folacin. Check labels because amounts vary.

TABLE 8-11   Protein

Food	Quantity	Protein (g)
Complete proteins		
Lentils	1 c*	30
Beef chuck roast	3 oz	28
Pork, center loin	3 oz	27
Turkey	3 oz	27
Chicken breast	3 oz	26
Flounder	3 oz	25
Tuna, canned	3 oz	24
Beef, lean ground	3 oz	22
Scallops	3 oz	16
Cottage cheese	½ c	15
Ham	3 oz	15
Eggs	2 lg	12
Shrimp	3 oz	11
Yogurt	1 c	8
Milk, any type	8 oz	8
Cheddar cheese	1 oz	7
Incomplete proteins		
Tofu	½ c	10
Green peas	1 c	9
Peanut butter	2 Tbsp	8
Egg noodles	1 c	7
Brown rice	1 c	5
White rice	1 c	4
Bread, whole wheat	1 slice	3

*Cooked

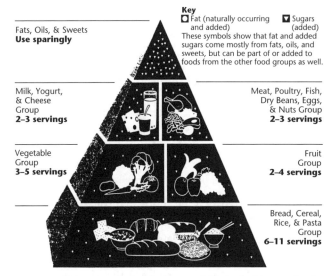

FIGURE 8-1 *Food Guide Pyramid: A Guide to Daily Food Choices.**

Source: U.S. Department of Agriculture/U.S. Department of Health and Human Services.

What Counts as One Serving?*

Breads, Cereals, Rice, and Pasta
  1 slice of bread
  ½ cup of cooked rice or pasta
  ½ cup of cooked cereal
  1 oz ready-to-eat cereal

Vegetables
  ½ cup of chopped raw or cooked vegetables
  1 cup of leafy raw vegetables

Fruits
  1 piece of fruit or melon wedge
  ¾ cup of juice
  ½ cup of canned fruit

Milk, Yogurt, and Cheese
1 cup of milk or yogurt
1½ to 2 oz cheese

Meat, Poultry, Fish, Dry Beans, Eggs, and Nuts
2½ to 3 oz cooked lean meat, poultry, or fish
Count ½ cup of cooked beans, or 1 egg, or 2 tablespoons of peanut butter as 1 oz of lean meat (about ⅓ of a serving)

Fats, Oils, and Sweets
Limit calories from these, especially if weight loss is needed

The amount eaten may be more than one serving. For example, a dinner portion of spaghetti would count as two or three servings of pasta.

How Many Servings Are Needed?
Teenage boys and active men need the highest number of servings shown. Women and some older adults need the lowest number of servings shown. Children, teenage girls, active women, and most men need a number of servings somewhere in the middle of those shown.

*Source: Human Nutrition Information Service. *Food Guide Pyramid: A Guide to Daily Food Choices.* Washington, DC: U.S. Department of Agriculture; 1992. Leaflet No. 572.

Notes

Chapter 9

Exercise During Pregnancy[1]

Management
1. Establish a database
   Motivation
   Exercise history and classification
   Nutritional status
2. Screen for
   Contraindications to exercise
   Conditions for assessment
   Conditions that may benefit from exercise
   Warning signs
3. Develop an exercise prescription
   Priorities and components of exercise
   Appropriate types of activities
   Special exercises for pregnancy
   Safety issues
4. Periodically assess and evaluate the exercise program
5. Evaluate in relationship to outcome

Safety Issues

Instructions for Pregnant Women

1. Be aware of theoretical concerns, such as the diversion of the uterine blood flow for exercise, the risk of hyperthermia, stress response and uterine irritability, and physical effects of vigorous motion.
2. Be aware of contraindications and warning signs.
3. Be aware of hypotensive syndromes.
4. Avoid fatigue, overtraining, and binge exercise.
5. Take in adequate calories at regular intervals.
6. Stay well hydrated and avoid hot, humid situations.
7. Be aware of safety in equipment and clothing.
8. If you are a professional dancer or competitive athlete, monitor your reactions and those of the fetus carefully.

Notes

Medical Screening

Name: Date:

Signature of care provider:

TO THE CARE PROVIDER: Please review these conditions and indicate if any now exist or existed previously. Please make any notes you think may be helpful. If any conditions that require assessment occur, please let us know. Thank you.

Contraindications for exercise:
__Placenta previa
__Premature rupture of membranes (PROM)
__Incompetent cervix
__Chronic heart disease
__Premature labor
__Toxemia
__Tearing or separation of placenta (abruptio)
__Fever (or presence of infection)
__Acute and/or chronic life-threatening condition

Conditions for assessment:
__Marginal or low-lying placenta
__History of IUGR
__Diabetes or hyperinsulinemia
__Irregular heart beat or mitral valve prolapse
__Anemia
__Multiple gestations
__Thyroid disease
__Three or more spontaneous abortions
__Excessive over- or underweight
__Extremely sedentary lifestyle
__Asthma

Conditions that may benefit from exercise:
__Diabetes
__Gestational diabetes
__Hyperinsulinemia
__Overweight
__Discomforts
__Depression
__Weakness
__Lack of stamina

Warning signs or symptoms:
__Edema of face and hands
__Severe headaches
__Hypertension
__Dizziness or disorientation
__Palpitations or chest pain
__Difficulty walking
__Nausea
__Bleeding or fluid discharge
__Regular strong contractions
__Cramps
__Fever

FIGURE 9-1   *Medical Screening Form for Prenatal Exercise Participants.*

Source: © 1985, 1995 Ann Cowlin. Used by permission.

TABLE 9-1 Prenatal Maternal Activity Chart

Activity	Inactive	A Little Active	Active	Very Active	Competitive or Professional
Walking	1 2 3	1 2 3	1 2 3	1 2 3	1 2 3
Speedwalking		2 3	1 2 3	1 2 3	1 2 3
Jogging*			1 2	1 2	1 2 3
Running*			1 2	1 2	1 2 3
Track events*			1	1 2	1 2
Treadmill*		1 2	1 2 3	1 2 3	1 2
Stair machine*		1 2	1 2	1 2 3	1 2 3
Slide§					
Glidewalker*‖				1 2	1
Stationary cycling	1 2	1 2	1 2 3	1 2 3	1 2
Recreational cycling*‖		1 2	1 2	1 2	1 2 3
Competitive cycling*‖					1 2
Recreational swimming*‖	1 2 3	1 2 3	1 2 3	1 2 3	1 2 3
Water aerobics	2	1 2 3	1 2 3	1 2 3	1 2 3
Lap swimming*			1 2 3	1 2 3	1 2 3
Competitive swimming*‖				1 2	1 2
Snorkeling*‖		1 2	1 2 3	1 2 3	1 2 3
Water skiing§					1 2
Scuba diving§					
Surfing§					
Day sailing*‖		1 2	1 2	1 2	1 2

(Continued)

TABLE 9-1 (Continued)

Activity	Inactive	A Little Active	Active	Very Active	Competitive or Professional
Sailboarding*‖					1
Rowing or sculling*‖				1 2	1 2 3
Ergometer rowing*			1 2	1 2 3	1 2 3
White water canoeing, kayaking§					
Prenatal aerobic/exercise class	1 2 3	1 2 3	1 2 3	1 2 3	1 2 3
Low-impact/low-intensity aerobics		1 2	1 2 3	1 2 3	1 2 3
Low-impact/high-intensity aerobics*			1 2	1 2 3	1 2 3
High-impact/high-intensity aerobics§					1
Low-step aerobics, beginning*		1 2	1 2 3	1 2 3	1 2 3
Low-step aerobics, advanced*‖			1 2	1 2 3	1 2 3
High-step aerobics, advanced*‖					1
Modern dance, beginning	1 2	1 2	1 2 3	1 2 3	1 2 3
Modern dance, advanced*			1 2	1 2 3	1 2 3
African/Caribbean dance, beginning		1 2	1 2 3	1 2 3	1 2 3
African/Caribbean dance, advanced			1	1 2	1 2
Ballet, beginning*		1 2	1 2 3	1 2 3	1 2 3
Ballet, advanced*			1 2	1 2	1 2 3
Jazz dance, beginning*			1 2	1 2	1 2
Jazz dance, advanced*‖			1	1 2	1 2

Activity					
Ballroom dance, beginning	1 2	1 2 3	1 2 3	1 2 3	1 2 3
Ballroom dance, advanced*‖			1 2	1 2 3	1 2 3
Contra dance		1 2 3	1 2 3	1 2 3	1 2 3
Gymnastics*‖	1 2 3			1	1
Prenatal yoga		1 2	1 2 3	1 2 3	1 2 3
Yoga, beginning*			1	1 2	1 2
Yoga, advanced*				1	1
T'ai chi	1 2	1 2	1 2 3	1 2 3	1 2 3
Karate, beginning*			1	1	1 2
Karate, advanced§					
Judo, beginning*			1	1	1 2
Judo, advanced§					
Badminton*	1 2	1 2	1 2 3	1 2 3	1 2 3
Basketball*‖			1	1 2	1 2
Frisbee*‖	1	1	1 2	1 2	1 2
Golf		1	1	1 2	1 2
Handball§					
Ping pong*			1 2	1 2	1 2
Racketball*‖			1	1	1
Soccer*‖			1	1	1
Softball*‖			1	1	1
Squash§					
Tennis*‖			1 2	1 2	1 2 3

(Continued)

TABLE 9-1   (Continued)

Activity	Inactive	A Little Active	Active	Very Active	Competitive or Professional
Volleyball*‖			1	1 2	1 2
Cross-country skiing*‖			1 2	1 2	1 2
Ski machine*‖			1	1	1
Downhill skiing§					
Snow or skate boarding§					
Roller skating or blading*‖			1	1 2	1 2
Ice skating*‖			1 2	1 2	1 2 3
Rock climbing*‖				1	1
Skydiving§					

Key: 1 = first trimester; 2 = second trimester; 3 = third trimester.

*Requires special skills and/or familiarity with equipment and poses dangers because of demands of those skills or equipment

‖Risky even with previous experience because the environment cannot be controlled; becomes increasingly dangerous as pregnancy progresses

§Not recommended for women in any stage of pregnancy

Reminder: The appropriateness of any activity is ultimately a matter that only the expectant mother herself can assess.

Source: © 1995 Ann Cowlin. Used by permission.

Chapter 10

Antepartal Complications[1]

Spontaneous Abortion[2]

Threatened Abortion

Signs and symptoms
- Vaginal bleeding: bright red (fresh) or dark brown (old)
- May be slight
- May be persistent for several days to 2 weeks
- Lower abdominal cramping or low backache

Management
1. First trimester with slight bleeding, without cramping
   - Bedrest has not been shown to be beneficial; normal activity may be continued unless the woman is uncomfortable or she prefers to rest
   - Pelvic rest (no intercourse, douching, or insertion of anything into vagina)
   - No sexual activity that causes orgasm

- Notify midwife immediately if there is
  - Increase in bleeding
  - Increased cramping or lower back pain
  - Gush of fluid from vagina
  - Fever or flu-like symptoms
- Examine on next day in office
  - Evaluate vital signs
  - Speculum exam—screen for vaginitis and cervicitis; observe cervix for opening, protrusion of membranes, clots, or fetal parts
  - Bimanual exam—uterine size, tenderness, effacement, dilatation, status of membranes Obtain hemoglobin and hematocrit, type & Rh (if not already available)
2. If exam is negative, ultrasound examination may be obtained to determine viability, dating, and to reassure the woman, if possible
3. If physical exam and ultrasound are negative, reassure woman, reiterate warning symptoms and keep normal appointments
4. If bleeding is heavy, cramps are increasing, or results of physical exam or ultrasound are abnormal, physician consultation is necessary

Inevitable Abortion
When spontaneous abortion (SAB) is almost certain by diagnosis of cervical dilatation, rupture of membranes, vaginal bleeding, cramping, and low back pain

Management
1. If the midwife has never seen the woman, refer to physician care
2. If the woman is the midwife's patient, assess the following
   - Gestational age
   - Amount of bleeding
   - Amount of abdominal pain

- Emotional status
- Previous or stat hematocrit
- Degree of dilatation
- Vital signs

Completion of the SAB may occur by D&C or at home, spontaneously. SAB may take place at home, if

- The woman desires it
- First trimester
- No excessive bleeding (bleeding soaks < one full-sized sanitary pad in 1 hour; no clots > 2 1/2 cm)
- No excessive pain
- Normal vital signs
- Previous hematocrit ≥ 30%
- No fever (take temp q4h, must be < 100°F)
- Preferably, she will not be alone
- If 2 or more SABs, save conceptus for genetic studies, if possible

Referral for suction D&C is necessary if

- Any parameters above are exceeded
- The woman prefers it
- The physician requires it

Follow-up

- Support grieving process
- Contraceptive counseling
- If 2 or more SABs, refer for genetic and endocrinologic counseling
- Evaluate for developmental anomalies of genital tract, i.e., bicornuate uterus
- Resume sexual activity in 2 to 4 weeks
- Follow-up office exam at 6 weeks postabortion

Missed Abortion
Fetus dies, but is retained for a prolonged time (weeks)

Signs & symptoms
- Normal early pregnancy signs and symptoms

- Vaginal spotting or bleeding, with or without cramping, may or may not occur at time of fetal death
- Fundal height ceases to grow or may became smaller
- Regression of mammary changes of pregnancy
- Loss of a few pounds of weight
- Persistent amenorrhea
- No fetal heart tones when expected

Management
1. Ultrasound exam for confirmation
2. Baseline coagulation studies
   - Prothrombin time
   - Partial prothrombin time
   - Fibrinogen level
   - Platelet count
3. Refer for physician consultation
4. Continued midwifery support

Follow-up
- Same as with inevitable abortion

Hydatidiform Mole[3]
- Degenerative process in placental chorionic villi causes development of cystlike clear vesicles resembling a bunch of grapes
- Complete mole—all vesicles, absence of fetus
- Partial mole—has vesicles with development of a nonviable fetus
- Usually benign neoplasm, may develop choriocarcinoma
- Increased incidence over age 45

Signs and Symptoms
- Apparently normal first trimester
- Persistent nausea and vomiting
- Uterine bleeding (spotting or severe) by 12 weeks

- Possible anemia
- Uterine size large for dates
- Shortness of breath
- Enlarged, tender ovaries (theca lutein cysts)
- No fetal heart tones
- No fetal activity
- No fetal parts on palpation
- Preeclampsia before 24 weeks

Diagnosis
- Ultrasound is diagnostic
- Very high or rapidly rising serum hCG after 100 days from the LMP

Management
- Referral to consulting physician

Ectopic Pregnancy[4]
When the pregnancy implants anywhere except in the endometrium of the uterus

Tubal Pregnancy
Accounts for 95% of ectopic pregnancies

Signs and Symptoms
Woman may or may not know she is pregnant
- Sharp, stabbing, tearing severe lower abdominal pain
- Hypotension or shock may develop
- Abdomen is tender; vaginal exam is quite painful
- Cervical motion pain
- Tender, boggy mass may be palpated in the adnexae
- Fullness in the posterior fornix may be caused by blood in the cul-de-sac
- Pain on inspiration or referred shoulder pain
- Uterus may be displaced
- Uterine lining (decidual cast) may be expelled
- Diarrhea or vomiting

Management

1. Laboratory tests
   * Serum hCG may be low for gestational age or negative urine pregnancy test may be negative
   * WBC may be normal or range to 30,000
   * Hemoglobin/hematocrit
   * Type and Rh/antibody screen
2. Ultrasound
3. Refer for physician management

Notes

Tuberculosis[5]

Screening Test

Screening tests detect hypersensitivity to the tuberculin protein. The test most commonly used is the Mantoux test, known as a PPD (purified protein derivative).

The Mantoux test consists of 0.1 ml of purified protein derivative (PPD) tuberculin containing 5 tuberculin units, administered intradermally in the forearm. The reaction to the PPD should be read 48 to 72 hours after injection. If a patient's reaction is not read until after 72 hours and it is negative, the test should be repeated. A positive reaction may be measurable up to 1 week after testing.* Reaction is the diameter of a palpable swelling (induration), measured in millimeters. Erythema is not included in the measurement. Tuberculin reactions are classified as positive according to risk factors, as follows*:

*From *Core Curriculum on Tuberculosis: What the Clinician Should Know,* 3rd ed. Atlanta: Centers for Disease Control and Prevention, 1994, pp 19–23.

1. *Induration ≥ 5 mm*
   - Person who is known to have or is suspected of having HIV infection
   - Person in close contact with a person who has infectious tuberculosis
   - Person whose chest x-ray is suggestive of previous tuberculosis with inadequate or no treatment
   - Intravenous drug abuser whose HIV status is unknown
2. *Induration ≥ 10 mm*
   - Foreign-born person from an area of the world where tuberculosis is common (e.g., Latin America, Africa, Asia)
   - Member of a high risk racial or ethnic group (e.g., Native American, African American, Hispanic, Asian, or Pacific Islander)

- Member of a medically underserved, low-income population
- Member of a group identified locally as having an increased prevalence of tuberculosis (e.g., homeless person, migrant farmworker)
- Resident of a homeless shelter or a long-term care facility
- Intravenous drug abuser who is known to be HIV-negative

3. *Induration ≥ 15 mm*
- Person with no known risk factors for tuberculosis

All pregnant women with a positive skin reaction should have a chest x-ray, and you should inform your consulting physician. The woman's abdomen should be shielded during the x-ray procedure.

Hepatitis[6]

Inflammation of the liver is caused by several viral infections identified as Hepatitis A, B, C, D, and E, which may be identified through history, physical exam, and laboratory data, as follows. Evidence or suspicion of maternal hepatitis should result in referral of the woman to the consulting physician. Hepatitis is a reportable condition, so each midwife should know the regulations for their state.

History
- Blood transfusion within the past year
- Previous hepatitis or jaundice
- Exposure to someone with hepatitis or jaundice
- Multiple sex partners
- Sex with a bisexual male
- Intravenous drug abuse
- Country of origin
- Occupation
- Symptoms (See Hepatitis A and B following)

- Hemophilia
- Need for dialysis

Physical Examination
- Tender, enlarged liver
- Enlarged spleen
- Jaundice (of sclerae or entire body)

Laboratory Evaluation
- Positive hepatitis screening test or identification of specific hepatitis antigens and antibodies
- Elevated results on liver function tests: AST (SGOT), ALT (SGPT), LDH, and bilirubin

Viral Hepatitis A
Most common form of hepatitis in the world

Route of transmission
- Fecal—oral

Most common source
- Contaminated water and food (especially shellfish)

Signs and Symptoms

COMMON
- "Flu-like" symptoms
- Anorexia
- Malaise
- Fatigue
- Weakness
- Nausea
- Low-grade fever

UNCOMMON
- Urticaria
- Arthritis
- Arthralgia
- Myalgia
- Jaundice
- Right upper quadrant abdominal or epigastric pain

- Enlarged and tender liver
- Pruritis
- Splenomegaly
- Muscle pain
- Weight loss

Course of disease
- Rapid onset
- Short acute phase of 10 to 15 days
- Symptoms resolved within 2 months
- No chronic or carrier state
- No known risk to newborn
- Vertical transmission has not been shown

Prophylaxis
- Family and close contacts should be given immune globulin (IG), previously known as immune serum globulin (ISG)
- Hepatitis screening is not necessary prior to receiving immune globulin (IG)

Viral Hepatitis B

Route of transmission
- Blood; blood by-products
- Contaminated needles
- Saliva
- Vaginal secretions
- Semen

Signs and symptoms
- Nausea, vomiting
- Right upper quadrant abdominal pain
- Enlarged and tender liver
- Fever, chills
- General weakness
- Exhaustion
- Headache

- Nonhepatic symptoms (rash, fever, arthralgia, myalgia, arthritis) generally precede jaundice

Course of disease

MATERNAL INFECTION
- Longer incubation than Hepatitis A
- May last 1 to 6 months
- May result in chronic or carrier state
- Increases risk for chronic active hepatitis, chronic liver disease, cirrhosis of the liver, and hepatocellular carcinoma
- Vertical transmission to the newborn is common

MATERNAL-NEWBORN TRANSFER
- Can occur at birth through contact with infected maternal blood
- May occur during close contact in early postpartum period
- May occur regardless of route of delivery
- Hepatitis B virus is present in all of an infected woman's body fluids, except in *breast milk*
- Breastfeeding is not contraindicated unless the woman has cracked or bleeding nipples or breast abscess

Prophylaxis for women
- ACOG and CDC recommend routine Hepatitis B virus screening for all pregnant women
- Women with negative results on screening should be considered for vaccination, if not already vaccinated
- Pregnancy is not a contraindication for Hepatitis B vaccine or Hepatitis B immune globulin HBIG

Prophylaxis for newborns of Hepatitis B–infected mothers
- Immediate bath after birth

- Should receive 0.5 ml HBIG (Hepatitis B immune globulin) IM within 1 hour of birth
- The baby should also receive Hepatitis B vaccine at birth and two or three more times in the first year
- Mothers who are HBeAg-positive at the time of birth are most likely to transmit the disease to the newborn

Precautions to Avoid Exposure to Hepatitis

In addition to standard (universal) precautions:

Antepartum
- Gloves on both hands and careful technique with speculum and bimanual examinations
- Careful handling of specimens (e.g., blood, urine, vaginal discharge)

Labor
- Careful technique when conducting vaginal examinations
- Careful disposal of used bed linens and Chux (wear gloves)
- Careful handling of bedpans, soiled Chux, and urine or stool specimens (wear gloves)
- No internal electronic fetal monitoring
- No scalp pH assessments

Delivery
- Protective eyeglasses
- Mask and gown
- Double gloves
- Careful delivery technique
- Careful handling of needles
- Careful disposal of linens

Postpartum
- Stool and blood precautions

Rubella[7]

Rubella antibody titer for immunity should be done, ideally, before pregnancy. It is also part of the initial antepartum visit.

Risk of Baby Being Born with Congenital Malformations

- If contracted in first trimester, 20% chance
- If contracted in first month, may be as high as 50%

Malformations Caused by Rubella

- Cataracts
- Cardiac defects
- Deafness
- Glaucoma
- Microcephaly
- Defects of eyes, ears, heart, brain, and central nervous system
- Severely affected fetuses may abort spontaneously

Antibody titer values

- 1:10 or above, immunity
- < 1:10, lack of immunity
- ≥ 1:64 may indicate present infection

Clinical Signs and Symptoms (Often Subclinical)

- Low-grade fever
- Drowsiness
- Sore throat
- Rash—pale or bright red, spreading rapidly from the face over the entire body, then fading rapidly
- Swollen neck glands
- Duration of 3 to 5 days

Management

If a woman is nonimmune and has a known or suspected exposure, obtain serologic testing (IgG and IgM) and consult physician.

Administration of Vaccine
- If nonimmune and not pregnant: give vaccine, advise against pregnancy for 3 months
- If nonimmune and pregnant: advise to avoid exposure during pregnancy and give vaccine during immediate postpartum period
- Vaccine is not contraindicated in breastfeeding
- If woman conceives within 3 months after receiving vaccine: no need for termination as no evidence of teratogenicity has been demonstrated

Varicella[8]
- Varicella (chickenpox) is a highly contagious form of herpesvirus
- Up to 95% of adults have a history of childhood varicella, which confers lifetime immunity
- 25% to 40% of exposed fetuses demonstrate congenital varicella syndrome (only if mother contracts the disease, not if she is just exposed)
- Greatest risk in first 20 weeks

Congenital Varicella Syndrome
- Cataracts
- Chorioretinitis
- Limb hypoplasia
- Hydronephrosis
- Microcephaly
- Mental retardation
- Dermatome lesions
- Cutaneous scars

Maternal Varicella Infection
- If occurs 6 days before to 2 days after delivery, can be passed to newborn
  - No time for mother to develop and pass on immunity
  - Infant may become seriously ill

- About 5% of infants who contract varicella around the time of birth die
- Varicella infection in adults leads to varicella pneumonia in 10% to 30% of cases
- In pregnancy, varicella pneumonia leads to maternal death in 40% of cases

Transmission
- Direct contact
- Respiratory transmission
- Incubation 10 to 21 days from exposure to first symptoms
- Communicable 2 days before lesions until all lesions are crusted over (7 to 10 days)
- Exposed or infected woman should be seen before or after regular office hours by staff known to be immune to varicella

Clinical Signs and Symptoms of Varicella Infection
- Fever
- Chills
- Myalgia
- Arthralgia
- Vesicles: pruritic, blister-like
- Lesions begin on head and neck; then spread to trunk and extremities; break open and crust over

Signs and Symptoms of Varicella Pneumonia
- Symptoms develop 1-6 days after vesicles appear
- Nonproductive cough
- Pleuritic chest pain
- Persistent fever
- Dyspnea

Vaccine
- Screen women during preconception visits; offer varicella serologic testing if a woman has no history of childhood infection

- Vaccine can be offered before pregnancy
- Contraindicated in pregnancy; avoid conception for 3 months after vaccine

Management of Care of Woman with Varicella Based on Patient Exposure or Route of Infection[9]

Household member exposed to varicella (e.g., child in day care)

1. Determine history of varicella in exposed household member.
2. Conduct serologic test for immunity in woman.
3. Have woman avoid contact with exposed household member until incubation period ends without evidence of infection.

Direct exposure to varicella (child with infection)

1. Conduct serologic test for immunity.
2. Administer VZIG within 96 hours of exposure if woman's immunity is negative or unknown.

Varicella infection in mother in first 20 weeks of pregnancy

1. Provide symptomatic relief with mild analgesics and antipyretics.
2. If woman is experiencing fulminant disease with high fever, extensive rash, and/or pulmonary symptoms, refer to physician for intravenous acyclovir.
3. Consult physician for ultrasound and possible fetal blood sampling (identify fetal infection).

Varicella infection in mother after 20 weeks but no later than 10 days before delivery

1. Provide symptomatic relief with mild analgesics and antipyretics.
2. If woman is experiencing fulminant disease with high fever, extensive rash, and/or pulmonary symptoms, refer to physician for intravenous acyclovir.
3. Infant will receive passive immunity from mother.

Varicella in mother beginning in the period 6 days before delivery

1. Give VZIG to mother.
2. Prepare for the possibility of tocolysis.
3. Give VZIG to infant at birth.
4. May need to isolate infant from mother, even if no maternal rash.
5. Possibly pump breast milk for infant, to minimize infant's contact with any maternal lesions.

Varicella in mother beginning within first 72 hours postpartum

1. Treat infant with VZIG.
2. Treat mother with VZIG if rash has not appeared (may reduce risk of serious infection).
3. Isolate mother and baby together.
4. Pump breast milk for infant, to minimize infant's contact with any maternal lesions.

Exposure of mother or baby to varicella after 72 hours postpartum

1. Determine serologic status of mother (immune mother passes antibodies to fetus/newborn).
2. Treat infant of nonimmune mother with VZIG or notify infant health care provider.
3. Avoid mother or baby contact with infected individual.

Urinary Tract Infections[10]

Presence of bacteria in urine is significant if a clean-catch specimen contains ≥ 50,000 bacteria of the same species/ml.

Contamination of a specimen is indicated, and woman should not be treated, when results are

- up to 100,000 nonpathogenic organisms/ml
- > 100,000 of mixed specis bacteria/ml

Repeat culture, if indicated

Table 10-1 Management of Urinary Tract Infections (UTI)

Diagnosis	Symptoms	Anticipated Lab Results	Treatment
Acute cystitis, first infection, uncomplicated	Dysuria, urgency, frequency, nocturia, suprapubic heaviness or discomfort; fever uncommon	Midstream voiding: WBCs, bacteriuria $>10^2$ to 10^5/ml dipstick: WBCs and nitrites	3 day Rx: TMP/SMX* 160 mg/800 mg, 1 DS tab bid; Nitrofurantoin (Macrodantin®) 100 mg bid; Amoxicillin 500 mg tid; first-generation cephalosporin, e.g. cephalexin (keflex) 500 mg qid
Asymptomatic bacteriuria	No symptoms, however increased incidence in women with history of: UTI's, diabetes, sickle cell trait	As above with positive culture	Pregnant women: Rx × 7 days as above** Non-pregnant women: Rx women with diabetes or sickle cell anemia: 7–10 days tetracycline 250–500 mg tid‖; Doxycycline 100 mg bid‖ Erythromycin 250 mg qid
Recurrent cystitis, >3/yr	Symptoms same as above, after sexual intercourse	Clean-catch voided specimen $>10^2$ to 10^5ml introital culture obtained at urethral meatus	Postcoital prophylaxis or single dose at bedtime for 6 mos. then repeat culture. Choose therapy based on sensitivity of bacteria responsible for preceding acute UTI; TMP/SMX, * 160 mg/800 mg 1 DS tab bid; nitrofurantoin 100 mg bid; cephalexin 500 mg bid

Interstitial cystitis	Frequency, urgency, often nocturnal; infra- and suprapubic pain; hematuria and hesi- tancy; generalized abdominal, back and rectal pain; pain with bladder filling and relief with emptying	Sterile urine, cytologically negative	Refer to physician for diagnosis by cytology, cystoscopy, +/or biopsy.
Acute pyelonephritis	Fever (102°F–105°F), malaise, back and flank pain; nausea and vomiting; urgency; frequency, dysuria; severe CVA tender- ness, usually unilateral	CBC with leukocy- tosis and left shift; UA with WBC's, bacteria $>10^2$ to 10^5 ml, urine culture positive	Consult physician; otherwise healthy, *non- pregnant* patients may be treated with outpatient therapy: 14 day course of Trimethoprim 100 mg bid; TMP/SMX* 160/800 1 DS tab bid; first-generation cephalosporin 500 mg qid; Amoxicillin 500 mg tid

*TMP/SMX:Trimethoprim/sulfamethoxazole (Bactrim®, Septra®) (Macrodantin) **do not use sulfonomides (TMP/SMX) or nitrofurantoin (Macrodantin) near term—2 weeks before EDD;
ᴵᴵcontraindicated in pregnancy and lactation.

Source: Adapted from the Sanford Guide to Antimicrobial Therapy, 1996.

Notes

Anemias and Hemoglobinopathies[11]

The working definition of anemia is generally accepted to be a hemoglobin level of less than 12.0 g/100 ml blood in nonpregnant women and less than 10.0 g/100 ml blood in pregnant women. Iron deficiency anemia constitutes approximately 95% of anemias related to pregnancy.

Anemia is generally asymptomatic in a woman with hematocrits above 30%, and in those with gradual onset. Symptoms commonly reported include

- Fatigue, drowsiness
- Dizziness, weakness
- Malaise
- Headache
- Sore tongue
- Poor appetite or anorexia
- Nausea and vomiting
- Loss of concentration

- Pica
- Shortness of breath (in severe anemia)

Findings on examination may include
- Skin pallor
- Pale mucosa, gums, and fingernail beds
- Tachycardia or flow murmur (in severe anemia)
- Brittle nails or hair (in severe anemia)
- Smooth tongue (in severe anemia)

TABLE 10-2 Laboratory Findings in Women with Anemia

Laboratory Test	Iron Deficiency	B$_{12}$ Deficiency	Folate Deficiency	Thalassemias	Chronic Disease
RBC	L	H	H	N	N
H & H	L	L	L	L	L
MCV	L	H	H	L	N–L
MCH	L	H	H	L	L
MCHC	L	N	N	L	N–L
Iron	L	H	H	H	L
TIBC	H	N	N	N	L
Ferritin	L	H	H	H	N–H

RBC = red blood cell count
H & H = hemoglobin level and hematocrit
MCV = mean corpuscular volume
MCH = mean corpuscular hemoglobin
MCHC = mean corpuscular hemoglobin concentration
TIBC = total iron-binding capacity
H = high; N = normal; L = low
N–L = normal to low
N–H = normal to high

TABLE 10-3   *Laboratory Tests, Diagnosis, Evaluation, and Management of Anemia[12]*

Laboratory Test	Laboratory Result/Interpretation	Management Additional Data Needed/Treatment
Hemoglobin	<10.0 g/dL; true anemia (hypochromic)	Management based on other indices
Reticulocyte count	Elevated above 2.5%; increased marrow activity due to blood loss or hemolysis	Review history for blood loss, hemolysis; order stool for ova and parasites
	Absent to low (<0.5%); marrow failure due to iron or folate deficiency or effect of medications	Review medications for risk of marrow depression side effect; change medication; supplement with iron and folic acid
Mean corpuscular hemoglobin (MCH)	Decreased; iron deficiency (hypochromic)	Supplement with iron
Mean corpuscular volume (MCV)	Low value MCV <80 μm³; iron deficiency (microcytic); confirms iron deficiency if serum ferritin is also low	Supplement with iron
	High value MCV >95 μm³; folate or vitamin B_{12} deficiency (macrocytic)	Order serum folate; if serum folate is low, supplement with folic acid;

Test	Results	Action
Serum iron	Elevated slightly; mobilization of iron stores	If serum folate is high or normal, consider vitamin B_{12} deficiency; Consult with physician for further evaluation; Supplement with iron
Serum ferritin	Low; depleted iron stores	Supplement with iron
	Elevated; iron overload, inflammatory diseases, alcoholism, inflammatory liver diseases	Consult physician for further evaluation
	Normal or elevated; chronic disease	Consult physician for further evaluation
Total iron-binding capacity (TIBC)	Low; iron stores depleted	Supplement with iron
	Elevated; response to fall in serum iron	Supplement with iron
Platelet count	Marked decrease; bone marrow depression; bone marrow failure (depends on extent of platelet decrease)	Consult physician for further evaluation
Hemoglobin electrophoresis	AA; normal	Inform woman
	AS; sickle cell trait carrier	Inform woman; monitor for urinary tract infections
	SS; sickle cell disease	Inform woman; consult physician for further evaluation and collaborative management

Women with a hemoglobin level between 10g/100ml (dL) and 12 g/100ml should be started on iron, folic acid, and vitamin supplements. They should also be counseled on high-iron foods (see p. 133), as iron is more readily absorbed from foodstuffs than from oral iron medication.

Possible Indications of Need for Consultation

- Initial hemoglobin below 9 gm/100ml
- Elevated MCV or Ferritin
- Decreased platelets
- Positive guaiac
- History of unexplained bleeding
- Failure to correct anemia with iron therapy

Glucose-6-Phosphate Dehydrogenase (G6PD) Deficiency

1. This x-linked genetic deficiency is common among those of Mediterranean and African ancestry.
2. Hemolysis can occur with infection, during surgery, and during therapy with antoxidant drug; also with ingestion of fava beans in Mediterranean women
3. Avoid these medications: sulfa, sulfa derivatives, nitrofurantoin (Macrodantin), toluidine blue, methylene blue.
4. If the woman's G6PD status is not known, a screen should be done before prescribing any of the above drugs, and the woman informed of the results and their interpretation.

Heart Disease[13]

Infection is of particular concern in a woman with cardiac disease because of the risk of developing bacterial endocarditis. Depending on the underlying disease, antibiotic prophylaxis may be recommended for labor and delivery or other invasive procedures during pregnancy.

Cardiac conditions associated with a *high* risk of endocarditis include:
- History of bacterial endocarditis
- Prosthetic cardiac valves
- Cyanotic congenital heart disease
- Pulmonary shunts or conduits

Cardiac conditions associated with a *moderate* risk of endocarditis include:
- Mitral valve prolapse with valvular regurgitation and/or thickened leaflets
- Congenital cardiac anomalies

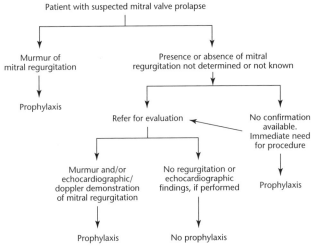

FIGURE 10-1 *Clinical Approach to Determination of the Need for Prophylaxis with Suspected Mitral Valve Prolapse.*

Evaluation = echocardiogram or doppler evaluation of the mitral valve.

Source: Adapted with permission from A.S. Dajani et al. Prevention of Bacterial Endocarditis. Recommendations by the American Heart Association. *JAMA,* June 11, 1997. 277(22):1794–1801. Copyright 1997. American Medical Association.

- Acquired valvular dysfunction (e.g., rheumatic heart disease)
- Hypertrophic cardiomyopathy

Cardiac conditions with a *minimal* risk of endocarditis include:

- Mitral valve prolapse without valvular regurgitation
- Physiologic, functional or innocent heart murmurs
- Isolated atrial septal defect
- Previous rheumatic heart disease without valvular dysfunction

TABLE 10-4   Clinical Consideration of Risk for Endocarditis

Clinical Consideration	Risk for Endocarditis		
	High	*Moderate*	*Minimal*
No evidence of infection:			
Prophylaxis	Optional	Not recommended	Not recommended
Known or suspected infection:			
Prophylaxis	Should be given	Should be given	Should be given

Genitourinary tract procedures for which prophylaxis should be considered

- Vaginal delivery
- Cesarean Section
- Urethral catheterization

- Uterine D&C
- Therapeutic abortion
- Sterilization procedures
- Insertion or removal of an IUD

TABLE 10-5 Recommended Prophylaxis for Genitourinary Procedures

Risk Status	Medication/Dosage
High	Initial dose within 30 min of starting procedure: Ampicillin 2 gm IM or IV; and Gentamycin 1.5 mg/kg (not to exceed 120 mg) IM or IV 6 hr later: Ampicillin (only)1 gm IM or IV
Moderate	2 hr before the procedure: Amoxicillin 2 gm orally *or* Within 30 min of procedure: Ampicillin 2 gm IM or IV
If Penicillin Allergic	
High	To be completed 30 min before procedure: Vancomycin 1 gm IV over 1–2 hr and Gentamycin 1.5 mg/kg (not to exceed 120 mg) IM or IV
Moderate	To be completed 30 min before procedure: Vancomycin 1 gm IV over 1–2 hr

Asthma[14]

- 1% to 4% of pregnant women are affected
- Clinical course during pregnancy is unpredictable
- Associated with
  - Increased perinatal mortality
  - Hyperemesis gravidarum

- Preterm delivery
- Chronic hypertension
- Preeclampsia
- Low birth weight
- Vaginal hemorrhage

  Management
- Avoid environmental factors that may exacerbate asthma
  - Allergens: Pollen, dust, soaps, pets
  - Over-the-counter medications: aspirin, ibuprofen
  - House-dust mites
- Medications commonly used are safe and effective in pregnancy
  - Inhaled bronchodilators (Proventil, Alupent, Brethaire)
  - Oral theophylline (Theo-Dur, Slo-Bid)
  - Anti-inflammatory agents: beclomethasone (Vanceril, Beclovent), flunisolide (Aerobid), and prednisone
- During labor and delivery to prevent bronchospasm
  - Continue regular medications
  - Maintain good hydration
  - Manage pain appropriately/avoid morphine and meperidine (Demerol)
- If prostaglandin is needed for postpartum hemorrhage
- Use prostaglandin E_2 (PGE_2) (dinoprostone)
- Prostaglandin F_2 alpha ($PGF_2\alpha$); Hemabate, Carboprost, or Prostin/15m may all trigger bronchospasm in women with asthma

Diabetes Mellitus[15]
Screen all pregnant women at 28 weeks gestation. If the screening test is normal, no further testing is needed. Risk factors indicating screens at first prenatal visit and at 28 weeks:

1. Family history of diabetes mellitus (parents, siblings, grandparents)
2. History of previous unexplained stillbirth
3. Poor obstetrical history (e.g., spontaneous abortions, congenital anomalies)
4. Previous delivery of newborn weighing 9 pounds or more
5. Nonpregnant weight greater than 180 pounds (may vary, depending on height and body build)
6. Recurrent monilial infections (if this condition occurs by itself, screen only at 28 weeks)
7. Recurrent glycosuria (two positive test results) in clean-catch specimens, not explained by dietary intake.
   If glycosuria occurs early in pregnancy and does not recur, do not repeat the screen later in pregnancy.
   Glycosuria secondary to dietary intake illustrates the lowered renal threshold for glucose, which is a normal physiologic change during pregnancy.
8. Signs and symptoms of diabetes:
   • Polyuria (excessive urine output)
   • Polydipsia (excessive thirst)
   • Polyphagia (excessive eating)
   • Weight loss
   • Poor healing
9. Preeclampsia or chronic hypertension
10. Polyhydramnios
11. Gestational diabetes in a previous pregnancy

A woman with secondary risk factors such as preeclampsia, polyhydramnios, or a large-for-gestational-age fetus should be screened when these risk factors are first noted, regardless of any previous screening with negative results.

A fasting plasma blood sugar of 105 mg or greater per 100 ml of blood, a 1-hr 50-g glucose challenge plasma blood sugar of 135 mg or greater per 100 ml of blood, and a 2-hr 75-g glucose challenge plasma blood sugar of 120 mg or greater per 100 ml of blood are abnormal values.

A 3-hr, 100g oral GTT is considered abnormal, or diagnostic for diabetes, if two or more of the following glucose values are met or exceeded:

Using whole blood with a glucometer (mg glucose/dl of whole blood):

Fasting—90 mg/dl (100 ml)
1 hr—165 mg/dl (100 ml)
2 hr—145 mg/dl (100 ml)
3 hr—125 mg/dl (100 ml)

Using plasma (most laboratory results: mg glucose/dl of plasma):

Fasting—105 mg/dl (100 ml)
1 hr—190 mg/dl (100 ml)
2 hr—165 mg/dl (100 ml)
3 hr—145 mg/dl (100 ml)

*TABLE 10-6   Management Plan for
            Diabetic Screening[16]*

Fasting Blood Sugar	+	1- or 2-hr Glucose Challenge	=	Indicated Action
Positive		Negative		Do GTT
Negative		Positive		Do GTT
Positive		Positive		Do *not* do GTT; the woman is diabetic. Consult physician.

TABLE 10-7 *Diagnoses Based on Laboratory Tests and Indicated Management*[17]

Fasting Blood Sugar	+	1- or 2-hr Glucose Challenge	+	Glucose Tolerance Test	=	Diagnosis	Management
Positive		Negative		Two abnormal values		Diabetic (probably requires insulin)	Collaborate with physician
Negative		Positive		Two abnormal values		Gestational diabetic	Consult with physician
Positive		Positive		Not done		Diabetic	Collaborate with physician
Negative		Negative		Not done		Not diabetic	Physician not needed

*Dietary Guidelines for Women With Gestational Diabetes (or Those at Risk)**

Avoid sugar and concentrated sweets
- No cookies, cakes, pies, soft drinks, chocolate, table sugar, fruit juices, fruit drinks, Kool-Aid, Hi-C, nectars, jams, or jellies
- Read labels: avoid foods containing sucrose, fructose, corn syrup, dextrose, honey, molasses, natural sweeteners, cornstarch, and concentrated fruit juices

Avoid convenience foods
- No instant noodles, canned soups, instant potatoes, frozen meals, or packaged stuffing

Eat small frequent meals
- Eat about every 3 hours
- Include a good source of protein at every meal and snack. High-protein foods are low-fat meat, chicken, fish, low-fat cheese, nuts, peanut butter, cottage cheese, eggs, and turkey

Eat a very small breakfast
- No more than one Starch/Bread exchange
- No fruit or juice
- Include a protein source and a dairy source

Choose high-fiber foods
- Whole-grain breads and cereals
- Fresh and frozen vegetables
- Beans and legumes
- Fresh fruits (except at breakfast)

Lower fat intake

- Buy lean protein foods: chicken, roast beef, turkey, ham, and fish. Limit lunch meat, bacon, sausage, and hot dogs
- Remove all visible fat: remove skin of poultry; trim fat from meat
- Bake, broil, steam, boil, or barbecue foods (no frying)
- Use nonstick pan, vegetable oil spray, or small amounts (1–2 tsp) of oil for cooking
- Use skim or low-fat (1%) milk and dairy products
- Eat boiled beans (not refried)
- Reduce added fat in the diet, such as butter, margarine, sour cream, mayonnaise, nuts, avocados, cream, cream cheese, or salad dressings

Free foods—eat as desired

  cabbage
  cucumbers
  green onions
  mushrooms
  zucchini
  spinach
  celery
  green beans
  radishes
  lettuce

*Source: Reprinted by permission from the American Diabetes Association. Medical Management of Pregnancy Complicated by Diabetes. Alexandria, VA: American Diabetes Association, Inc. 1993.

Thyroid Disease

Hypothyroidism

Signs and symptoms

  Bradycardia
  Hypothermia
  Dry, cold skin

Hoarseness
Delayed DTR relaxation
Diastolic hypertension
Menorrhagia
Fatigue
Cold intolerance
Weight gain
Constipation
Muscle cramps
Weakness
Depression

Hyperthyroidism

Signs and symptoms
Tachycardia
Tremor
Hyperkinesis
Weight loss
Nervousness
Oligomenorrhea
Goiter
Palpitations
Heat intolerance
Shakiness
Frequent stools
Insomnia
Warm, moist skin
Exopthalmos

Hypertensive Disorders of Pregnancy[18]

Definitions

1. Preeclampsia—development of an elevated blood pressure *with* proteinuria due to pregnancy; primarily a complication of primigravidas, occurring after 20 to 24 weeks gestation except in the presence of trophoblastic disease

2. Eclampsia—preeclampsia plus one or more convulsions

3. Chronic hypertensive vascular or renal disease with or without superimposed preeclampsia or eclampsia

4. Gestational hypertension (pregnancy-induced hypertension, or PIH)—the development of an elevated blood pressure *without* proteinuria during pregnancy or within the first 24 hr postpartum in a previously normotensive woman who has no evidence of hypertensive vascular disease

5. Gestational proteinuria—the presence of proteinuria *without* coexisting hypertension during pregnancy, with no evidence of any urinary tract infection or history of intrinsic renovascular disease

6. Gestational edema—the development of a *general* and excessive accumulation of fluid in the tissues (measured as greater than 1+ pitting edema after 12 hr rest in bed) *without* coexisting hypertension or proteinuria

Preeclampsia

The classic clinical signs of preeclampsia are the triad of hypertension, proteinuria, and edema. These three clinical signs are defined as follows:

1. Hypertension
   a. blood pressure of 140/90 or higher, or
   b. a rise of 30 mm Hg in the systolic pressure and/or rise of 15 mm Hg in the diastolic pressure over the woman's baseline blood pressure, or
   c. mean arterial pressure equal to or more than 105 mm Hg for two readings taken 6 hr apart
      (1) in reality, the second reading is often taken the next day

(2) mean arterial pressure is calculated as follows:

$$MAP = \frac{(D \times 2) + S}{3}$$

where MAP = mean arterial pressure
 D = diastolic blood pressure
 S = systolic blood pressure

2. Proteinuria
   a. protein in the urine at a concentration of more than 0.3 g in a 24-hr specimen, or
   b. protein in the urine in excess of 1 g/L(1+ to 2+)
      (1) in random clean-catch, midstream voided specimen, and
      (2) on two or more occasions at least 6 hr apart when there is no known urinary tract infection
3. Edema
   a. fluid retention first evidenced by a sudden excessive weight gain (2 to 5 lb or more in a week)
   b. differentiated from dependent edema in the lower extremities
   c. evaluated in relation to the overall pattern of weight gain
   d. unquestionably significant when in the hands and face

Associated or Predisposing Conditions to Preeclampsia
1. Trophoblastic disease—occurs in up to 70% of women with hydatidiform mole; occurs prior to 24 weeks gestation
2. Multiple pregnancy—greater for primigravidas although also increases for multiparas; overall the incidence is approximately 30%
3. Chronic hypertensive vascular disease—20% incidence
4. Chronic renal disease

5. Diabetes mellitus—approximately 50% incidence
6. Fetal hydrops—approximately 50% incidence; occurs in early pregnancy
7. Maternal age greater than 35
8. Nulliparity
9. Familial tendency—a woman has double the risk of developing preeclampsia if her mother had preeclampsia; a one-in-four chance of developing preeclampsia if her mother had eclampsia; and a significantly greater risk of developing preeclampsia if her sister had preeclampsia
10. Previous history of preeclampsia—one third develop hypertension (although not necessarily preeclampsia) in a subsequent pregnancy

Preeclampsia screening on each prenatal visit:
1. History
   a. headaches, dizziness, blurring of vision, spots before the eyes, or scotomata
   b. hand, face, or general body edema
2. Physical examination
   a. blood pressure (compare to baseline blood pressure either before pregnancy or prior to 24 weeks gestation)
   b. weight (compare to prepregnant weight and to weight at last visit; note visit interval)
   c. ankle, pretibial, hand, face, or abdominal edema (note amount)
   d. reflexes (note degree of reflex response)
3. Laboratory test
   a. urine for protein

For women whose symptoms are suggestive of preeclampsia, but not yet diagnostic, the midwife may prescribe: 1) bedrest—at least 2 hr in the morning and afternoon on her left side, and 2) a high protein, high calorie diet. Limitation of salt intake or use of diuretics are *not* indicated in the prevention or management of preeclampsia.

Evaluation of Symptoms

A history of unremitting headaches and visual problems, elevated blood pressure, sudden excessive weight gain, hand or face edema, proteinuria, or a combination of any of these indicates the need for further investigation, as follows:

1. History
   a. rule out migraine headaches, need for glasses, and stress and tension in the woman's personal life
   b. evaluation of dietary intake (see Chapter 8)
   c. evaluation of the overall weight gain pattern
2. Physical examination
   a. ophthalmic examination—papilledema, A-V nicking, vessel narrowing, hemorrhagic areas
3. Laboratory tests (see Table 10-8 on pp. 188–189):
   a. hemoglobin and hematocrit
   b. platelet count
   c. liver function tests
   d. kidney profile
      (1) BUN
      (2) serum creatinine and creatinine clearance
      (3) serum uric acid
   e. urine protein
   f. coagulation profile

Severe Preeclampsia

Signs and symptoms of progressively severe preeclampsia, when associated with hypertension, proteinuria, or edema, include the following:

1. Hyperreflexia (extremely severe when clonus is present)

2. Headaches (frontal or occipital); usually resistant to customary effective treatment
3. Visual disturbances—blurring of vision, scotomata, flashing lights, spots before the eyes
4. Epigastric pain
5. Oliguria—less than 500 cc in 24 hr
6. Increasingly elevated blood pressure; 160/110 and above is considered severe
7. Increasingly greater proteinuria; 3+ or 4+ is considered severe
8. Increasingly severe hand, face, or generalized body edema

Progressive preeclampsia may result in development of the HELLP syndrome, which stands for Hemolysis; Elevated Liver enzymes; and Low Platelets. A woman with HELLP syndrome may not exhibit hypertension or renal changes usually associated with preeclampsia.

Collaborative management in the hospital may include:

1. Bedrest
2. Decreased environmental stimulation
3. Screening for diabetes
4. Ruling out multiple pregnancy
5. 24-hr record of intake and output
6. High protein, high calorie diet
7. Monitoring of liver and kidney function
8. Evaluation for uteroplacental insufficiency and assessment for possible IUGR with ultrasound if the woman is earlier than 36 weeks
9. Evaluate fetal well-being: FMC, NST, BPP or CST
10. Magnesium sulfate infusion

TABLE 10-8   *Interpretation of Laboratory Findings in Preeclampsia*[19]

Laboratory Test	Finding	Interpretation	Comment
Hemoglobin and hematocrit	Increased	Hemoconcentration	Fluid moves from intravascular to extracellular, causing edema
Platelet count	Decreased	Cause unknown	Falling platelets indicate progressive disease <100,000 platelets is severe disease
Serum uric acid	Increased	Reflects severity of preeclampsia Decreased renal clearance	Serum uric acid increases as renal excretion of uric acid decreases
Blood urea nitrogen (BUN)	Normal	Mild preeclampsia	Doubling of BUN represents 50% reduction in renal blood flow
	Increased	Decrease in renal blood flow and glomerular filtration rate indicates increasing severity of preeclampsia	
Serum creatinine	Normal	Mild preeclampsia	Doubling of serum creatinine represents 50% reduction in renal blood flow
	Increased	Decrease in renal blood flow and glomerular filtration rate indicates increasing severity of preeclampsia	
Creatinine clearance	Decreased	May be normal in less severe preeclampsia; is decreased in severe preeclampsia	More useful measure than a single serum creatinine value
Liver function tests:	Elevated	Liver cell damage	Serious complication of preeclampsia is subcapsular hemorrhage in the liver

LDH (lactate dehydrogenase)		Indicates severe disease
AST (SGOT)—serum glutamic oxalacetic transaminase		
ALT (SGPT)—serum glutamic pyruvic transaminase		
Coagulation profile:		Measures blood clotting ability; abnormal clotting function is indicative of severe disease
Fibrinogen	Low	
Fibrin split products	Present	
PT—prothrombin time	Prolonged	
PPT—partial prothrombin time	Prolonged	
Urine protein (dipstick)	Increased	3+ and 4+ in severe disease
Urine protein (24-hour)	Increased protein	Renal compromise with increased permeability	2+ indicates need for 24 hr collection; 300 mg in 24 hr, or 1 g/L in preeclampsia; 5 g/L in 24 hr in severe disease
	Decreased urine volume	Hypovolemia, hypoperfusion, renal compromise	Less than 400–500 ml in 24 hr in severe disease

11. Evaluation for timing of delivery based on:
    a. severity of preeclampsia
    b. fetal well-being
    c. gestational age

Chronic Hypertension

Women with chronic hypertension must be scrutinized for development of superimposed preeclampsia. Any indication of proteinuria or an increase in blood pressure above the woman's normal values should be carefully evaluated to rule out preeclampsia. A baseline set of liver and renal function studies, a diabetes screen, and a careful ophthalmic examination should be obtained early in pregnancy.

Eclampsia

Diagnosed when preeclampsia progresses to seizures.

- Most common prior to delivery
- May occur up to 10 days postpartum

   PREMONITORY SIGNS:
- Severe headache
- Visual disturbances
- Epigastric or right upper quadrant pain
- Restlessness

   EMERGENCY MANAGEMENT OF ECLAMPTIC SEIZURE
   (*NOTHING WILL STOP THE CURRENT SEIZURE*)

1. Call for help and consultant physician *stat*
2. Observe the seizure—do not attempt to stop or control it
3. Note length of seizure, nature of seizure, e.g., tonic-clonic vs. focal
4. Prevent injury:
    a. Use side rails
    b. Turn to side to prevent aspiration

c. Do not attempt to restrain, except to keep in bed or from falling

If possible, attempt to place an airway or tongue blade *only* very early in the seizure, not after the seizure is in progress

5. Prepare to initiate magnesium sulfate for prevention of further seizures

IMMEDIATE MANAGEMENT AFTER THE SEIZURE

1. Establish intravenous line
2. Administer IV magnesium sulfate; usual dose is a 4–6 g bolus given at l g/min followed by a maintenance dose
3. Clear the airway, suction thoroughly
4. Maintain airway and suction until the woman regains consciousness
5. Administer oxygen per face mask at 8 L/min
6. Initiate fetal monitoring to evaluate fetal status. The fetus will have had a hypoxic episode, and may have severe bradycardia during the seizure, rebounding with tachycardia. A compromised fetus may not be able to tolerate the hypoxic episode and therefore continue with bradycardia, severe tachycardia of > 200 bpm, and/or late decelerations.
7. Evaluate uterine contractions and labor status
8. Examine the woman for injury
9. Evaluate maternal blood gases, electrolytes, hematologic status, coagulation factors, and magnesium level

DELIVERY CONSIDERATIONS

- Labor often becomes rapidly progressive
- The mother must be stabilized prior to induction or cesarean delivery

Intensive nursing care and medical management is required to prevent intracranial hemorrhage, pulmonary edema, renal damage, and retinal detachment.

Notes

Antepartal Bleeding[20]

Placenta Previa

Implantation of the placenta in the lower uterine segment, either partially or completely covering the internal cervical os. This may be a serious cause of antepartum hemorrhage in the third trimester or in labor.

Predisposing conditions

- Multiparity
- Maternal age > 35
- Multiple pregnancy
- Erythroblastosis
- Previous uterine surgery, including cesarean section
- Smoking
- Previous placenta previa
- Previous therapeutic abortion

Signs and symptoms

- Painless bleeding or hemorrhage with sudden onset
- May be accompanied or precipitated by uterine irritability

Management

When placenta previa is suspected due to a bleeding episode:

- *Do not* do a vaginal examination until there is a definitive diagnosis
- Sonography should be performed to confirm exact placental location
- Evaluate fetal well being
- If bleeding is severe initiate an intravenous line (see page 196)
- If the woman is at term and in labor, a cesarean section must be performed. If she is in preterm labor, the risk benefit ratio between tocolysis and delivery is considered, unless there is uncontrollable hemorrhage
- If the woman has a total placenta previa, she is hospitalized for the remainder of her pregnancy

- If the woman has a partial or marginal placenta previa, is not delivered, and the bleeding resolves, she may be discharged to home with:
  - Reduced activity, sometimes complete bedrest
  - Pelvic rest (nothing in vagina; no orgasmic activity; no vaginal therapeutics)
  - 24-hour plan for emergency transport
  - Immediate telephone access
  - Weekly NST or BPP
- If the woman is Rh-negative, Rh immune globulin should be administered if the woman remains undelivered. A Kleihauer-Betke test may be useful to determine the dosage needed.

Abruptio Placentae

When there is premature separation of a normally implanted placenta, hemorrhage may be from the placental margin or within the mass of the placenta. Therefore, bleeding may be obvious or concealed.

Associated factors

- Maternal hypertension
- Preeclampsia
- Folic acid deficiency
- Severe abdominal trauma
- Short umbilical cord
- Malnutrition
- Sudden decrease in uterine volume or size, e.g., rupture of the membranes in polyhydramnios, delivery of a first twin
- Maternal age over 35
- Rough or difficult external version
- Cocaine, especially "crack" cocaine, usage

Signs and symptoms

May differ between anterior and posterior placental implantation, and will vary dependent upon the degree of separation

- Board-like uterus (may not occur, especially if placenta is located on the posterior wall)
- Severe, unrelenting abdominal pain
- Back pain
- Colicky, discoordinate uterine activity interspersed with relaxation of the uterus
- Contractions may be hypertonic
- Bleeding may be concealed or obvious; therefore, the total amount of blood loss may be difficult to appreciate except by symptoms
- Woman's pain is out of proportion to what the examiner feels
- Painful localized or generalized uterine tenderness
- Fetal heart rate (FHR) pattern may be normal or with late or variable decelerations, loss of short-term variability, or sinusoidal
- Fetal movement may be very aggressive immediately after a large abruption or may be very decreased if the abruption is smaller, but causes fetal distress. If the abruption has been severe, cessation of fetal movement and fetal death occurs rapidly.
- Concealed hemorrhage may cause a rising fundal height.
- Maternal shock may occur with a massive hemorrhage.
- Ultrasound may identify a retroplacental clot. However, a negative ultrasound examination cannot rule out abruptio placentae.

Management
- Delivery
- If woman is stable and there is evidence of fetal well-being, vaginal delivery may be attempted with rupture of membranes, internal fetal monitoring, and pitocin induction or stimulation, if indicated.
- In emergent situations, cesarean section is indicated.

Management of Hemorrhage in Placenta Previa and Abruptio Placentae

Management of a woman who is hemorrhaging, either from placenta previa or abruptio placentae, is the same and consists of the following:

1. Call for help and request that your physician consultant be notified.
2. Start 5% dextrose in Ringer's lactate intravenously with a 16-gauge intracatheter.
3. When starting the IV, obtain blood for type and cross-match for three or more units, CBC, platelets, PT, PTT, fibrinogen, and a tube for clotting time to hang on the wall.
4. Place the woman in Trendelenburg position.
5. Monitor the woman's vital signs (blood pressure, pulse).
6. Monitor the fetal heart tones with an external monitor.
7. Administer oxygen to the woman.
8. Cover the woman with warm blankets.
9. Start a second IV. Two intravenous infusion routes are needed: one for electrolyte solutions and the other for blood transfusion. Keep the IV line for blood transfusion open until the blood is obtained.
10. Have the operating room set up for an emergency cesarean section.
11. Insert a Foley catheter to measure output and in preparation for possible surgery.

ABO and Rh Disease[21]

All women should have laboratory evaluation of blood type, Rh and antibody screen (indirect Coombs') at the first prenatal visit.

If woman is Rh-positive and antibody screen is negative: no further evaluation is necessary.

If woman is Rh-negative and antibody screen (indirect Coombs') is negative:

- Repeat indirect Coombs' test at 28 weeks
- If negative for antibodies at 28 weeks, offer 300 mcg Rh immune globulin
- If more than 12 weeks pass and the woman is undelivered, offer another dose of 300 mcg Rh immune globulin
- Reassess antibody titers on admission to labor and delivery

    if titer < 8 of anti-D—passive immunity present from Rh immune globulin

    if titer > 8—suggests active immunization due to Rh incompatibility

If the indirect Coombs' (antibody screen) is positive at any time

- Obtain Rh antibody titers
- Consult with physician

Nonroutine uses of antepartum Rh immune globulin

- After spontaneous or elective abortion
- After amniocentesis or chorionic villus sampling
- After trauma to maternal abdomen, i.e., car accident, fall, domestic violence
- After vaginal bleeding indicative of abruption or placenta previa

Size-Dates Discrepancy[22]

When you suspect a size-dates discrepancy, differential diagnosis is necessary in order to determine the cause of this discrepancy. Possibilities include:

1. Erroneous dates
2. Large baby (size greater than expected for dates)
3. Intrauterine growth retardation (size smaller than expected for dates)

4. Multiple pregnancy (size greater than expected for dates)
5. Diabetes:
   a. gestational to class B (size greater than expected for dates due to a macrosomic infant)
   b. classes C and above (size smaller than expected for dates)
6. Thyroid disease (size smaller than expected for dates)
7. Inadequate nutritional intake or inadequate weight gain pattern (size smaller than expected for dates)
8. Polyhydramnios (size greater than expected for dates)
9. Oligohydramnios (size smaller than expected for dates)
10. Fetal lie:
    a. transverse lie or oblique lie (size smaller than expected for dates)
    b. breech presentation—longitudinal lie (size greater than expected for dates)
11. Congenital anomalies
12. Station of presenting part (size smaller than expected for dates, if the presenting part is deep in the pelvis)
13. Hypertension or preeclampsia
14. Psychosocial factors—for example, death in family, severe emotional shock
15. Viral infection such as toxoplasmosis, rubella, cytomegalic inclusion disease
16. Chemical dependency, including tobacco, alcohol, illicit drugs (size smaller than expected for dates)
17. Placenta previa (size greater than expected for dates, if fetus is in a longitudinal lie; size smaller than expected for dates, if fetus is in a transverse lie)
18. Uterine fibroids (size greater than expected for dates)

Intrauterine Growth Restriction/Small for Gestational Age[23]

Intrauterine Growth Restriction (IUGR)
- Impaired or restricted fetal growth
- Pathological process
- Strongly related to diminished oxygen/nutritional availability to the fetus

Risk factors
- Poor nutrition
- Poor maternal weight gain
- Prepregnancy weight < 90 lbs
- Maternal vascular disease
- Heart disease
- Preeclampsia
- Renal disease
- Maternal viral or bacterial infection
- Genetic abnormalities
- Multiple gestation
- History of previous IUGR pregnancy
- Illicit substance abuse
- Smoking
- Alcohol abuse
- Anemia
- Diabetes (class C or greater)
- Hypoglycemia
- Late onset of prenatal care
- Low socioeconomic status

Small for Gestational Age (SGA)
May also reflect:

- Constitutionally small fetus
- Not pathological

Diagnosis
It is difficult, if not impossible, to differentiate IUGR from SGA fetuses before birth.

- Serial ultrasound examinations are necessary to establish gestational age and then to follow growth patterns of the fetus.
- Serial scans must be at least 3 weeks apart to be diagnostic.
- Evaluation of fetal size and growth is based on measurement of biparietal diameter, abdominal circumference, and femur length.
- A fetal growth curve less than expected or flattening (lack of progressive growth) is indicative of IUGR.
- Decreased amniotic fluid volume is highly associated with hypoxia and IUGR.

Management

- Serial ultrasound examinations to follow fetal growth
- Serial fetal assessment to evaluate fetal well-being
- Screen for underlying medical complications, e.g., hypertension, diabetes, preeclampsia, anemia, renal disease
- No smoking, no alcohol, no illicit substances
- Limit maternal activity; increase rest periods, periods of bedrest in left lateral position
- Improve nutritional status: high-protein, high-calorie diet
- Have pediatrics alerted prior to delivery as there is an increased risk for meconium aspiration, hypoglycemia, hypocalcemia, and polycythemia
- Reduction of household and job responsibilities

Hydramnios (Polyhydramnios)[24]

Polyhydramnios is an excessive amount of amniotic fluid. Women with the following conditions exhibit a higher incidence of polyhydramnios:

- Multiple pregnancy (especially monozygotic twins)
- Uncontrolled gestational diabetes

- Erythroblastosis
- Fetal malformations, especially of the gastrointestinal tract, e.g., TE fistula, or CNS, e.g., anencephaly, meningomyelocele
- Chromosomal abnormality

Hydramnios may produce the following further complications:

- Fetal malpresentations
- Premature separation of the placenta (abruptio)
- Uterine dysfunction during labor
- Immediate postpartum hemorrhage as a result of uterine atony from overdistention
- Cord prolapse
- Preterm labor

The signs and symptoms of polyhydramnios include:

- Uterine enlargement, abdominal girth, and fundal height far beyond that expected for gestational age
- Tenseness of the uterine wall, making it difficult or impossible to
    Auscultate fetal heart tones
    Palpate the fetal outline and large and small parts
- Elicitation of a uterine fluid thrill
- Mechanical problems, if polyhydramnios is severe, such as
    Severe dyspnea
    Lower extremity and vulvar edema
    Pressure pains in the back, abdomen, and thighs
    Nausea and vomiting
- Frequent change in lie (unstable lie)

If you suspect that a woman has polyhydramnios, the following work-up should be done:

- Obtain an ultrasound to confirm the diagnosis and identify any coexisting conditions or complications

- Screen for diabetes
- Screen for ABO/Rh disease

Oligohydramnios[25]

Oligohydramnios is an abnormally small amount of amniotic fluid, which is associated with a marked increase in perinatal mortality. Women with the following conditions have a higher incidence of oligohydramnios:

- Congenital anomalies (e.g., renal agenesis, Potter's syndrome)
- Intrauterine growth retardation
- Early rupture of the fetal membranes (24 to 26 wks)
- Postmaturity syndrome

Longstanding oligohydramnios may lead to the complications of lung hypoplasia or limb deformities in the fetus.

The clinical signs and symptoms of oligohydramnios include:

- "Molding" of the uterus around the fetus
- A fetus that is easily outlined
- A fetus that is not ballotable
- Lagging fundal height

Amniotic fluid volume is measured by ultrasound and is a standard component of the biophysical profile.

Discussion with the consulting physician should include identification of the underlying etiology of the oligohydramnios and consideration of different management strategies based on etiology and gestational age.

Conservative management includes

- Bed rest
- Hydration

- Good nutrition
- Monitor fetal well-being (fetal movement counts, NSTs, BPP)
- Regular ultrasound measurement of amniotic fluid volume
- Amnioinfusion
- Induction and delivery

Postdates Pregnancy[26]

Postdates Pregnancy

When pregnancy exceeds 42 weeks (294 days) from the first day of the last menstrual period.

Postmaturity Syndrome

Postdates pregnancy accompanied by:

- Oligohydramnios
- Meconium-stained amniotic fluid
- Newborn with:
  - Loss of subcutaneous fat
  - Long fingernails
  - Wrinkled peeling skin
  - Alert facies
  - Absence of lanugo
  - Absence of vernix caseosa

Management

Fetal surveillance includes

- Fetal movement counting
- NST twice weekly beginning by 41 weeks *and* amniotic fluid volume measurement twice weekly *or*
- BPP weekly from 41 weeks, with twice weekly amniotic fluid volume

Delivery Indications

- Any nonreassuring tests of fetal surveillance:
  - Nonreactive NST

- Oligohydramnios
- BPP ≤ 6 with **normal** amniotic fluid volume
- Positive CST
- Decreased fetal movement
- If the cervix is ripe at 42 weeks, induction should be considered
- Physician consultation is recommended after 42 weeks

Notes

Chapter 11

Intrapartum[1]

Diagnosis of Labor and Initial Evaluation

History to be reviewed or obtained at onset of labor:

Maternal Age

- Less than 16 years, increased risk of toxemia
- More than 35 years, increased risk of chronic hypertension, gestational diabetes, ectopic pregnancy, prolonged nulliparous labor, cesarean section, preterm delivery, IUGR, chromosomal abnormalities, fetal death

Gravida/Para

- Affects duration of labor
  - Primigravidas have longer labor
  - Multiparas have shorter labors
  - Grand multiparas may have prolonged labors
- Affects rate of complications: multiparas have increased risks of:
  - Placental abruption
  - Placenta previa
  - Postpartum hemorrhage
  - Perinatal and maternal mortality
  - Double ovum twinning

Method of Previous Deliveries
- Previous cesarean section
- Previous midforceps deliveries

Size of Previous Babies
- Assures adequacy of pelvis up to size of largest baby born vaginally
- Helps rule out IUGR
- May assist in determination of route of delivery for breech fetus

EDD and Current Gestational Age
- Determines term vs. preterm status
- Determines SGA/AGA/LGA fetal size vs. gestational age

History of Present Pregnancy
- Essential to evaluate obstetrical risk factors
- Obtain most recent laboratory values
  - Blood type/Rh antibody screen
  - Hemoglobin/hematocrit
  - Hepatitis screen/syphilis screen/STD cultures
  - Pap smear
  - Rubella immunity
  - Group B beta-hemolytic streptococci
  - MSAFP/triple screen
  - Genetic screening
- Current medications or medical treatments
- Obtain ultrasound reports from pregnancy
- Evaluate course of pregnancy
  - Blood pressure changes
  - Growth of fundal height
  - Weight gain

Last Oral Intake
- Determine nutritional/hydration status
- Evaluate presence of nausea/vomiting

Past Obstetric History
- Note history of incompetent cervix/cerclage

- Note previous obstetrical surgery
  - Previous classical cesarean section
  - Previous low transverse cesarean section
  - Previous multiple abortions or miscarriages

Past Medical and Primary Health Care History
- Note chronic medical problems
- Note previous surgery that may have effect on labor/birth
  - Previous myomectomy entering uterine cavity
  - Multiple previous abdominal surgeries
  - Previous cervical conization
- Note drug allergies
- History of blood transfusion and any reactions
- Note previous anesthesia reactions

Family History (Obtain or Review)
- Pertinent medical or genetic history

Specific History for Diagnosis of Labor:

Time of onset, frequency and duration of contractions*
- Important to establish start of labor
- Differentiate true/false labor

Intensity of contractions; lying down vs. walking*
- Differentiate between true/false labor
- True labor intensifies with walking
- False labor rarely intensifies with walking, may feel relief

Description of location of pain with contractions*
- Differentiate between true/false labor
- True labor felt as radiating across the uterus from the fundus to the back
- True labor has progressively more intense/painful contractions
- False labor felt throughout uterus, especially in middle to lower portion and groin

Length of previous labor*
- A good indicator of the potential length of this labor, allowing for differences between a primigravid and a secundigravid labor as well as anticipation of changes for grandmultiparas

Number of years since last birth*
- If more than 10 years since last birth, labor may be prolonged

Presence of bloody show*
- Premonitory sign of labor
- Increase in bloody show suggests impending second stage

Presence of vaginal bleeding*
- Abnormal finding
- Contraindication to vaginal examination
- May indicate need for sonogram to rule out placenta previa
- Frank bleeding requires physician consultation

Status of membranes*
- Ruptured membranes are a premonitory sign of labor
- Document approximate time of rupture
- Document color of amniotic fluid if membranes are ruptured

Assess fetal movement*
- Indication of fetal well-being

*Pertains to evaluation of labor status.

Physical Assessment at Onset of Labor
(Obtain or Review):

General observations and screening physical examination
- Update baseline data
- Screen for current infection
- Screen for symptoms of labor

Vital signs
- To determine initial status and establish baselines for duration of labor and birth
- Elevated systolic BP with normal diastolic may indicate anxiety

Weight
- May be performed to determine total weight gain
- May be used to help evaluate severity of edema with preeclampsia

Assessment of fetal well-being
- Auscultation of fetal heart tones
- May require electronic fetal monitoring (EFM)
- May require assessment of amniotic fluid volume
- Fetal movement

Contraction pattern*
- Frequency of contractions
- Duration of contractions
- Intensity of contractions

Abdominal scars
- Obtain explanation for any scars

Engagement*
- Determine by abdominal palpation
  If unengaged in primigravida may indicate CPD
  - Reevaluate clinical pelvimetry and closely observe progress of labor

Estimated fetal weight and fundal height*
- If fetus seems > 4000 grams or larger than previous infant, carefully assess pelvis and progress of labor to be prepared for possible shoulder dystocia

Abdominal girth, when indicated
- Screening for an oversized uterus
  - Twins or greater
  - Polyhydramnios

Lie, presentation, position, and variety*
- Ascertain fetal lie (transverse; longitudinal)
- Ascertain fetal presentation (cephalic, breech, shoulder)
- Ascertain fetal position and variety (occiput, sinciput, brow, mentum)
- Confirm with ultrasound if Leopold maneuvers are not diagnostic, or if they indicate an abnormal presentation for labor

Edema of the extremities
- Ankle, pretibial, finger, facial
- Evaluate for preeclampsia

Reflexes and clonus
- Hyperreflexia (3+, 4+), associated with severe preeclampsia
- Clonus often associated with eclampsia

Pelvic Examination at Onset of Labor:

Effacement and dilatation*
- Determine progressive cervical change
- Diagnose labor
- Determine stage/phase of labor

Position of the cervix*
- Indicates readiness for labor

Bloody show*
- Sign of impending second stage

Station*
- Determine descent of the presenting part of the fetus
- Indicative of labor progress
- Indicative of pelvic adequacy

Molding and caput succedaneum*
- Assess pressure on baby's head
- Extensive caput or molding may be indicative of CPD

Synclitism/asynclitism*
- Assess fetal adaptation to the pelvis

Lie, presentation, position, variety*
- Confirm abdominal examination
- Palpate presenting part to clarify fetal presentation/position/variety

Status of membranes*
- Examine for confirmation of rupture: ferning, positive nitrazine, gross rupture
- Note color of amniotic fluid
- Obtain culture, if indicated
- Assess fetal heart tones

Evaluation of vaginal orifice and perineal body
- Evaluate distensibility and length
- Observe for herpetic lesion, if woman has a positive history

Evaluation of bony pelvis, including clinical pelvimetry
- Assess pelvic adequacy

*Pertains to evaluation of labor status.

Intrapartal Laboratory Tests
May vary from setting to setting.

- Hematocrit
- Type, antibody screen (if indicated), and, for women at very high risk, i.e., grand multiparas, anemia, overdistended uterus, cesarean section, Rh-negative, bleeding, history of postpartum hemorrhage, consider crossmatch
- Urinalysis (minimum of dipstick for protein, glucose, and ketones)
- Review prenatal record for laboratory results

Signs and Symptoms of Impending Labor[2]
1. Lightening (approximately 2 wk before labor)
2. Cervical changes yielding "ripeness"

3. False labor (may go on for days or weeks)
4. Premature rupture of the fetal membranes (80% of women begin labor spontaneously within 24 hr)
5. Bloody show (labor usually occurs within 24 to 48 hr)
6. Energy spurt (approximately 24 to 48 hr before onset of labor)
7. Gastrointestinal upsets of no known cause may be indicative of impending labor

Progress in Labor According to Friedman

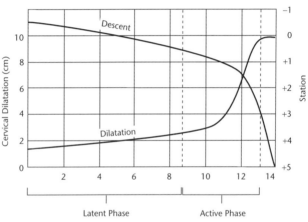

FIGURE 11-1   Nulliparous Dilatation and Descent.
Source: Adapted with permission from E. A. Friedman. An objective method of evaluating labor. *Hospital Practice* 5(7):82, 1970. © 1970 The McGraw-Hill Companies, Inc. Illustration by Albert Miller.

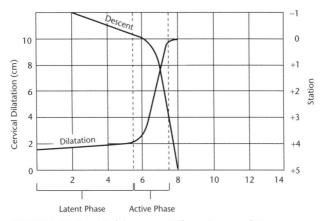

FIGURE 11-2   Multiparous Dilatation and Descent.
Source: Adapted with permission from E. A. Freidman. An objective method of evaluating labor. *Hospital Practice,* 5(7):82, 1970. © 1970 The McGraw-Hill Companies, Inc. Illustration by Albert Miller.

TABLE 11-1   General Course of Labor

	First Stage/ Phase		Second Stage	
	Latent (hr)	*Active (hr)*	*(hr)*	*Rate of Dilation (cm/hr)*
Nullipara				
Mean	6.4	4.6	1.1	3.0
Upper limit of normal	20.1	11.7	2.9	1.2
Multipara				
Mean	4.8	2.4	0.39	5.7
Upper limit of normal	13.6	5.2	1.1	1.5

Source: Adapted from E. A. Friedman. *Labor Clinical Evaluation and Management,* 2nd ed. New York: Appleton-Century-Crofts, 1978, p. 49.

Lie, Presentation, Position, and Variety[3]

Lie is the relationship of the long axis of the fetus to the long axis of the mother.

Presentation is determined by the presenting part, which is the first portion of the fetus to enter the pelvic inlet.

Position is the arbitrarily chosen point on the fetus for each presentation in relation to the left or right side of the mother's pelvis.

Variety is the same arbitrarily chosen point on the fetus used in defining position in relation to the anterior, transverse, or posterior portion of the pelvis.

Table 11-2 summarizes the possibilities.

Notes

TABLE 11-2   Possible Fetal Relationships to the Maternal Pelvis for Each Lie and Presentation[4]

Lie/ Presentation	Position*	Position and Variety‖	
Longitudinal			
Cephalic			
Vertex	Occiput	ROA	LOA
		ROT	LOT
		ROP	LOP
Sincipital	Sinciput (bregma, anterior fontanel)	Sinciput and brow presentations usually convert to either a vertex or a face presentation.	
Brow	Brow		
Face	Mentum (chin)	RMA	LMA
		RMT	LMT
		RMP	LMP
Breech			
Frank	Sacrum	RSA	LSA
		RST	LST
		RSP	LSP
Full	Sacrum	Same as frank presentation	
Footling	Sacrum	Same as frank presentation	
Transverse			
Shoulder	Acromion	RAA	LAA
		RAP	LAP
		A transverse variety is not possible.	

Oblique

With an oblique lie, the midwife will feel nothing at the inlet. There is no presentation, position, or variety associated with an oblique lie, which is usually a transitory condition.

---

*Arbitrarily chosen point on the fetus.

‖Designation for position (left or right side) and variety (anterior, transverse, or posterior portion of the mother's pelvis).

Mechanisms of Labor[5]

There are eight basic positional movements that take place when the fetus is in a cephalic vertex presentation.

1. Engagement
2. Descent
3. Flexion
4. Internal rotation _____ ° to the _____ position
5. Birth of the head by _____
6. Restitution 45° to the _____ position
7. External rotation 45° to the _____ position
8. Birth of the shoulders and body by lateral flexion via the curve of Carus

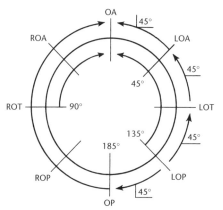

FIGURE 11-3   Degrees of Internal Rotation.[6]

Occiput Anterior

The mechanisms of labor for a fetus that begins labor in the LOA, LOT, LOP, ROA, ROT, or ROP position and delivers in an occiput anterior position are as follows:

1. Engagement takes place for LOT and ROT positions with the sagittal suture of the fetus in the transverse diameter of the pelvic inlet and the biparietal diameter of the fetus in the anteroposterior diameter of the pelvic inlet. For LOA, ROA, LOP, and ROP positions, engagement of the fetal head takes place with the sagittal suture in one of the oblique diameters of the pelvis (the right oblique diameter for LOA and ROP positions, and the left oblique diameter for ROA and LOP positions). The biparietal diameter is thus in the oblique diameter of the pelvis opposite from the one the sagittal suture is in. The sagittal suture is used as the fetal landmark that determines in which oblique diameter the fetal head is entering the pelvis.

2. Descent occurs throughout.

3. Flexion substitutes the suboccipitobregmatic diameter for the diameter that entered the pelvic inlet.

4. Internal rotation takes place:
    45° (for LOA and ROA positions)
    90° (for LOT and ROT positions)
    135° (for LOP and ROP positions—long arc rotation)

The fetal head is now in an occiput-anterior position in the anteroposterior diameter of the mother's pelvis.

5. Birth of the head by extension

6. Restitution 45° to the LOA or ROA position: the fetal head moves left if it started the mechanisms of labor with the occiput in the left side of the pelvis and right if it started the mechanisms of labor with the occiput in the right side of the pelvis.

7. External rotation 45° to the LOT or ROT position: the direction of the rotation of the shoulders is determined by the direction of restitution. External rotation brings the bisacromial diameter of the shoulders into the anteroposterior diameter of the maternal pelvis.

8. Birth of the shoulders and body by lateral flexion via the curve of Carus

Persistent Posterior

A persistent posterior position occurs when a right or left occiput posterior position undergoes internal rotation through a short arc of 45° to a direct occiput posterior position instead of a long arc rotation of 135° to a direct occiput anterior position. Short arc rotation is much less common, occurring approximately 6% to 10% of the time, most frequently in conjunction with an anthropoid or android type of pelvis.

The mechanisms of labor for a fetus that begins in the LOP or ROP positions and delivers in an occiput posterior position are the same as for those that rotate to an occiput anterior position, except as noted and explained below:

1. Engagement takes place in the right oblique diameter for the ROP position and in the left oblique diameter for the LOP position.
2. Descent occurs throughout.
3. Flexion
4. Internal rotation takes place: The fetal head rotates 45° to an occiput posterior position in the anteroposterior diameter of the mother's pelvis.
5. Birth of the head is by the double mechanism of flexion and then extension. The sinciput impinges beneath the symphysis pubis and becomes the pivotal point for delivery of the head. The head stays flexed as the occiput distends the perineum and is born to the nape of the neck. The remainder of the head is then born by extension, starting with the anterior fontanel and ending with the chin, as the head falls back toward the rectum with the face looking upward.

6. Restitution: The fetal head rotates 45° to the LOP or ROP position, depending on whether internal rotation was from the LOP or ROP position.
7. External rotation: The fetal head rotates 45° to the LOT or ROT position.
8. Birth of the shoulders and body by lateral flexion via the curve of Carus

Synclitism and Asynclitism[7]

Synclitism and asynclitism describe the relationship of the sagittal suture of the fetal head to the symphysis pubis and the sacrum of the mother's pelvis. *Synclitism* occurs when the sagittal suture is midway between the symphysis pubis and the sacral promontory. In *asynclitism*, the sagittal suture is directed either toward the symphysis pubis or toward the sacral promontory. Determination of whether this is anterior asynclitism or posterior asynclitism is based on which parietal bone is dominant.

In normal labor, the head usually enters the pelvic inlet with a moderate degree of posterior asynclitism and then changes to anterior asynclitism as it descends

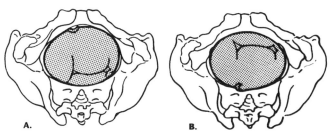

FIGURE 11-4   Asynclitism.
A. Anterior; B. Posterior.[8]

further into the pelvis before the mechanism of internal rotation takes place. This sequential change from posterior to anterior asynclitism facilitates the mechanism of descent; it is an accommodation by the fetus to take advantage of the roomiest portions of the true pelvis.

Notes

Management Plan for the Normal First Stage of Labor[9]

Management of the first stage of labor includes the diagnosis of labor, management of false labor, management of early labor, and the initial evaluation of the mother and fetus. Thereafter, midwifery management of care during the first stage of labor includes responsibility for the following, all of which may be going on simultaneously:

1. Continuing evaluation of maternal well-being
2. Continuing evaluation of fetal well-being
3. Continuing evaluation of the progress of labor
4. Bodily care of the woman
5. Supportive care of the woman and her significant other/family
6. Continuing screening for maternal or fetal complications
7. The 11 basic management decisions

The 11 basic management decisions are the decisions that routinely may be made about each woman in labor and individualized for that woman. Some of these decisions are relevant to a hospital setting and are not an issue if the woman is giving birth at home or in a freestanding out-of-hospital birth center.

1. Whether the woman is to have an IV
2. Whether the woman has any position or ambulation limitations
3. Whether the woman may have food or fluids by mouth
4. Whether to give the woman medication
5. The frequency with which the woman's vital signs (blood pressure, pulse, and temperature) are to be checked

6. The frequency with which the fetal heart tones are to be checked and how this will be done
7. The frequency with which vaginal examinations are done
8. Identification of the woman's significant others and their roles
9. Whether to artificially rupture the membranes and, if so, when
10. Determination of when there is a need for physician consultation or collaboration
11. When to prepare for delivery

Management Plan for the Second Stage of Labor[10]

1. Continuing evaluation of maternal well-being
2. Continuing evaluation of fetal well-being
3. Continuing evaluation of the progress of labor
4. Bodily care of the woman
5. Supportive care of the woman and her significant others and family
6. Continuing screening for signs and symptoms of maternal and fetal complications

In addition, the management of the second stage of labor includes these responsibilities:

7. Preparation for delivery
8. Management of the delivery

Second-stage management decisions include the following:

1. **Frequency** of woman's vital signs (blood pressure, pulse, and temperature)
2. **Frequency** of fetal heart tone checks
3. **Whether** to encourage the woman's pushing effort
4. **Location** of the delivery
5. **When** to prepare for delivery
6. **Position** of the woman for the delivery

7. Whether to catheterize the woman immediately before delivery
8. Whether to support the perineum and, if so, how
9. Whether to cut an episiotomy
10. If the decision is to cut an episiotomy, what type to cut
11. Type of analgesia/anesthesia
12. Whether to deliver the baby's head with a contraction or between contractions
13. Whether to use a Ritgen maneuver
14. Method of infant suction/resuscitation
15. When to clamp and cut the umbilical cord
16. Whether there is a need for physician consultation or collaboration

Second Stage Evaluation of Maternal Well-Being

Continuing evaluation of maternal well-being during the second stage of labor includes the items used to evaluate the first stage of labor.

1. Vital signs: blood pressure, temperature, pulse, and respirations
2. Bladder
3. Urine: protein and ketones
4. Hydration: fluids, nausea or vomiting, and perspiration*
5. General condition: fatigue and physical depletion, behavior and response to labor, and pain and coping ability
6. Maternal pushing effort*
7. Need for analgesia or anesthesia
8. Perineal integrity*

*Additional items specific to the second stage of labor.

Management of the Delivery

Management of the delivery includes using the proper hand maneuvers to assist the baby's birth and providing immediate care of the newborn. In managing the delivery, the midwife must decide the following:

1. Whether to deliver the baby's head with a contraction or between contractions
2. Whether to use a Ritgen maneuver
3. Method of infant suction/resuscitation
4. When to clamp and cut the umbilical cord

Indications for Intravenous Infusion[11]

1. Gravida 5 or greater
2. An overdistended uterus for any reason, including multiple gestation, polyhydramnios, and an excessively large baby (estimated at 9 lb or more)
3. An induction or augmentation with pitocin
4. History of previous postpartum hemorrhage
5. History or presence of any other condition that predisposes the woman to immediate postpartal hemorrhage
6. Maternal dehydration or exhaustion
7. Use of regional anesthesia
8. Any obstetric or medical condition that is life threatening, such as abruptio placentae, placenta previa, ruptured uterus, preeclampsia, or eclampsia

The usual intravenous solution for a woman in labor consists of 1000 cc D_5W or $D_50.2NS$ or D_5RL given at 125 cc per hour.

Fetal Monitoring in Labor[12]

- Baseline rate: 120 to 160 beats per minute (bpm), determined over 10 minutes
- Periodic changes: fetal heart rate (FHR) changes, associated with uterine contractions
- Short-term variability: beat-to-beat variation from the baseline
- Long-term variability: rhythmic fluctuation at 3 to 5 cycles per minute

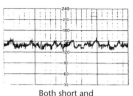

Both short and
long-term variability

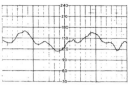

Long-term variability,
absence of short-term variability

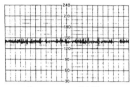

Short-term variability,
absence of long-term variability

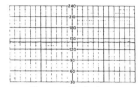

Absence of both short
and long-term variability

FIGURE 11-5   *Variations in Short-term and Long-term Variability.*

Source: Reproduced by permission from S. M. Tucker. *Pocket Guide to Fetal Monitoring,* 3rd ed. St. Louis: Mosby Year Book, 1996, p. 72.

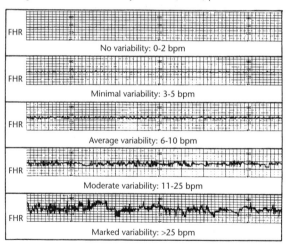

FIGURE 11-6   *Classification of Baseline Variability. Short-term and Long-term Variability Tend to Increase and Decrease Together.*

Source: Reproduced by permission from S. M. Tucker. *Pocket Guide to Fetal Monitoring,* 3rd ed. St. Louis: Mosby Year Book, 1996, p. 74.

Method of Assessment of FHR and Contractions

Documentation of a Fetal Monitor Strip Should Include:

1. Fetal heart
   - Baseline rate
   - Variability
   - Periodic changes
   - Response to fetal movement or stimulation
2. Contractions
   - Frequency
   - Duration
   - Intensity
3. Method of assessment
   a. Fetal heart tones
      Auscultation (fetoscope; doppler ultrasound)
      External fetal monitoring (tocodynomometer)
      Internal fetal monitoring (fetal scalp electrode)
   b. Contractions
      Palpation
      External fetal monitoring (tocodynomometer)
      Internal fetal monitoring (intrauterine pressure catheter [IUPC])

Auscultation of The Fetal Heart in Labor:

Appropriate for healthy women with uncomplicated pregnancy; evaluate through and after a contraction to assess periodic changes.

Standard frequency: Every 30 minutes in active labor, every 5 to 15 minutes in second stage.

Additional auscultation is done: at ROM, after an enema, with marked changes in contraction or labor pattern, at the time medication is given and at the time of peak effect, with any indication of medical or obstetrical complication.

Evaluation of Intrauterine Pressure:

Necessary if labor is nonprogressive and contraction strength is an issue.

TABLE 11-3   Medications Commonly Given in Labor[13]

Generic Name (Trade Name)	Class	Pain Relief	Decrease Anxiety	Sedation	Anti-emetic	Dosage & Route	When to Give
meperidine (Demerol)	Narcotic analgesic	x				50–75 mg IM q3–4h; 12.5–25 mg IV q2–3h	Active labor
nalbuphine (Nubain)	Synthetic narcotic agonist-antagonist analgesic	x		x		10–20 mg SQ or IM or IV q3–6h	Active labor
promethazine (Phenergan)	Ataractic, narcotic potentiator		x	x	x	25–50 mg IM or IV q4–6h	Early or active labor
butorphanol (Stadol)	Synthetic opioid agonist-antagonist analgesic	x		x		0.5–2 mg IV or 1–4 mg IM q3–4h	Active labor
hydroxyzine (Vistaril)	Ataractic, narcotic potentiator		x	x	x	25–100 mg IM (only) q4–6h	Early or active labor
morphine	Narcotic	x		x		10–15 mg IM q3–4h or 8–10 mg IV q2–3h	Prodromal labor, prolonged latent phase or hypertonic uterine dysfunction
secobarbital (Seconal)	Barbiturate, sedative		x	x		100 mg po or IM q3–4h	False/early labor
pentobarbital (Nembutal)	Barbiturate, sedative		x	x		100 mg po or IM	False/early labor

After inserting an IUPC, evaluate contractions for adequacy with Montevideo units (MVU).

Calculate MVU by subtracting the baseline uterine pressure from the amplitude of each contraction in a 10 min period and adding the results.

Diagnosis of arrest of active first stage labor is made when there have been $\geq$ 200 MVU in a 10 min period for 2 hr without cervical change.

Support and Comfort Measures in Labor[14]

Supportive care throughout labor is a hallmark of midwifery. Supportive care can miraculously change the entire scenario of a labor. It has both emotional and physiological positive effects on the mother and fetus, which may lead to less need for medication and intervention and even to a shorter labor.

5 Needs of a Laboring Woman (Lesser & Keane)
- Bodily or physical care
- Sustaining human presence
- Relief from pain
- Acceptance of her attitudes and behavior
- Information and reassurance of a safe outcome

Source: M. S. Lesser and V. R. Keane. *Nurse-Patient Relationships in a Hospital Maternity Service.* St. Louis: Mosby, 1956.

Guidelines for How to Provide Support
- Each woman responds differently and has different needs—ask her if a particular measure is helpful or desirable
- Define your purpose; what you are trying to accomplish with your support and comfort measures
- Speak to a laboring woman in a tone and manner that she can hear and interpret through stresses of labor
- Be involved with and/or facilitate the involvement of others—constant presence is necessary to real support

- Be realistic in your expectations of what you can accomplish with your support and comfort measures; each woman comes to labor with her own expectations, fears, pain threshold, preparation, personality, and behavioral makeup

Support and Comfort Measures

Positioning
- Use of pillows, rolled blankets, or towels to maximize relaxation
- Eliminate pressure points

Relaxation exercises
- Progressive relaxation
- Controlled relaxation
- Deep breath and sigh after each contraction

Breathing exercises
- Ideally learned before labor begins, but simple patterns may also be taught during labor
- Support and facilitate whatever method she has learned, practiced, or believes in
- She may need encouragement and clarification
- May need to be done by midwife simultaneously with the laboring woman

Prevention of exhaustion and provision of rest
- Use breathing techniques appropriate for each stage of labor
- Organize necessary procedures to cause the least disruption to the woman
- Control the environment to enhance a sense of restfulness, i.e., lighting, music, external noises, temperature, and people in the room
- Control the people in the room; consider effect of talking, conversation with or around the woman, effect of family, visitors, and hospital staff
- Focus should be on the woman and anything that facilitates efforts to cope and work with labor

Assurance of privacy and prevention of exposure
- Especially in hospital
- Especially concerning extra staff and students
- Respect each woman's need or lack of need for clothing and draping during labor and birth

Explanation of the process and progress of labor
- Explanation reduces fear of the unknown
- Alleviation of fear decreases the pain resulting from tension caused by fear

Explanation of procedures and imposed limitations
- Allows the woman to feel safe and cope effectively

Keeping clean and dry
- Promotes comfort and relaxation
- Decreases risk of infection
- Bath or shower can be very refreshing and relaxing

Tub bath/Jacuzzi
- Needs to be deep enough to cover the abdomen
- May be the most relaxing and facilitative comfort measure for labor

Mouth care
- Have woman brush teeth
- Mouthwash
- Glycerin swabs
- Lip petroleum
- Oral fluids

Usefulness of a washcloth
- Cleansing
- Cool compress to face and other body parts
- Warm compress to back
- Moisten lips or mouth
- Fanning

Fanning
- Fan with washcloth
- Fan with glove package
- Fan with her gown

Back rub
- General back massage
- OB back rub—firm pressure on the lower back for relief of pain related to a posterior presentation

Heat or cold to the lower back
- Promotes relaxation and pain relief

Abdominal rub
- Usually performed by a birth attendant
- Light strokes on abdomen
- Comforting

Effleurage ("feather touch")
- Done by the laboring woman
- Psychological influence—distracts attention
- Physiologic influence—encourages relaxation, increases circulation

Heat to the lower abdomen
- Decreases pain
- Increases circulation

Empty bladder
- Decreases abdominal pain
- Full bladder may slow labor, increase urine stasis, increase risk of bladder infection, cause pain

Medication
- Judicious use of medication constitutes a support and comfort measure (see p. 227)

Cold compresses
- To axilla and groin may bring relief and calm

Support during vaginal examinations
- Empty the bladder
- Explain reasons for examination
- Position woman comfortably
- Assist in relaxation and breathing during examination
- Super-gentle verbal and physical approach

- Warning if discomfort should be expected
- Explanation of findings

Alleviation of leg cramps
- Straighten leg and place foot in dorsiflexion
- Alternate dorsiflexion with relaxation of the leg (do not point toes)
- Do not massage cramp (to avoid possibility of dislodging a thrombus)

Use of physical touch
- Perceived differently by each woman; observe for reaction and response
- May be excellent means of communicating care and concern
- Good means of soothing, calming, and dispelling loneliness

Significant others
- May include spouse, partner, parents, children, close family, or friends
- May be the most therapeutic measure for many women
- Care must be taken to help the woman select persons who will actually be helpful to her
- Avoid family or friends who may cause tension for the woman with their presence
- Midwife should facilitate relationship(s) with the support person(s)

"Alternative" Comfort Measures

These measures use special skills that the midwife may learn to provide supportive care in labor. They are best taught to the woman before labor. All of these methods can be helpful in promoting relaxation, diminishing pain, and decreasing the need for intervention.

- Accupressure
- Therapeutic touch
- Visualization

- Therapeutic massage
- Hypnosis

The Third Stage of Labor

Signs of Placental Separation[15]

1. Sudden trickle or small gush of blood
2. Lengthening of the umbilical cord visible at the vaginal introitus
3. Change in the shape of the uterus from discoid to globular as the uterus now contracts on itself
4. Change in the position of the uterus: It rises in the abdomen because the bulk of the placenta in the lower uterine segment or upper vaginal vault displaces the uterus upward

Placenta and Cord Variations[16]

Succenturiate placenta

A succenturiate placenta occurs when one or more separate accessory lobes are in the membranes a variable distance away from the main placental mass. These accessory lobes are usually connected to the main placental mass by blood vessels extending out from the main placental mass. When there are no connecting blood vessels, the anomaly is called *placenta spuria*.

Manual exploration of the uterus and removal of the succenturiate lobe(s) is indicated if retention has occurred.

Extrachorial placenta

Extrachorial placenta is a placental anomaly observed on the fetal surface as a thick, white ring, which gives the impression that the central portion of the placenta is somewhat depressed. Within this depression the fetal surface looks as usual with the insertion of the umbilical cord. However, all the large blood vessels pass into the depths of the placenta before reaching the ring, instead of coursing over the totality of the fetal surface as they usually do.

There are two varieties of extrachorial placenta, which are determined by the location of the ring. Both may be complete or incomplete, as dictated by whether the ring circumscribes a full circle:

1. In placenta circumvallata (circumvallate placenta), the ring is situated a variable distance between the margin and the middle of the placenta.

2. In placenta marginata (circummarginate placenta), the ring is located at the edge, or margin, of the placenta.

Battledore placenta

Battledore placenta is a variation in which the umbilical cord inserts in the edge, or margin, of the placenta.

Velamentous cord insertion

Velamentous insertion is when the blood vessels in the umbilical cord separate and leave the cord before insertion into the surface of the placenta.

Vasa previa

Vasa previa occurs when unprotected blood vessels between the chorion and the amnion present first at the cervical os by crossing the os ahead of the fetal presenting part. May occur with velamentous cord insertion or with succenturiate placenta.

Notes

Chapter 12

Intrapartal[1] *Complications*

Cervical Ripening and Induction of Labor

Indications

- Premature rupture of the membranes
  - If maternal body temperature is rising
  - At term with positive group B beta-hemolytic streptococcus culture
  - When the management plan is to impose a limited number of hours before delivery
- Oligohydramnios
- Chorioamnionitis
- Post dates > 42 weeks
- Severe preeclampsia or pregnancy-induced hypertension
- Maternal diabetes mellitus—gestational or insulin-dependent
- Maternal medical complications
- Nonreassuring fetal testing (NST, CST, BPP)
- Fetal demise

Contraindications to Induction of Labor
- Cephalopelvic disproportion (CPD)
- Transverse lie
- Presenting part above the pelvic inlet
- Fetal distress/nonreassuring FHR pattern
- Cord presentation
- Placenta previa
- Unexplained vaginal bleeding
- Vasa previa
- Previous classical c/s or fundal uterine incision
- Active genital herpes infection
- Invasive cervical carcinoma

There is a direct correlation between the condition of the cervix and the success or failure of induction of labor.

Bishop's Score
The Bishop score is the total of the scores for each factor listed in Table 12-1. A maximum Bishop score of 13

TABLE 12-1 *Bishop Pelvic Scoring System for Evaluating Cervical Readiness for Induction or Need for Preinduction Cervical Ripening*

Factor	Score (points)			
	0	1	2	3
Dilatation (cm)	0	1–2	3–4	5–6
Effacement (%)	0–30	40–50	60–70	80
Station	–3	–2	–1/0	+1/+2
Consistency	Firm	Medium	Soft	
Position	Posterior	Mid	Anterior	

Source: E. H. Bishop. Reprinted by permission from the American College of Obstetricians and Gynecologists *Obstetrics and Gynecology* 1964; 24(2):267.

is possible. A score of at least 6 is likely to result in a successful labor induction. In general, cervical ripening is unnecessary with a Bishop score greater than 8.

Methods of Cervical Ripening and Induction of Labor

- Nipple stimulation

Use breast stimulation CST guidelines. Monitor FHR with auscultation or electronic fetal monitoring. Observe for hyperstimulation of the uterus.

- Sexual intercourse

Use only with intact membranes. Female orgasm causes uterine contractions. Semen contains prostaglandins.

- Castor oil

Use with a "ripe" cervix, especially for multiparas. One to 2 oz castor oil may be mixed with or followed by orange juice or other drink the woman prefers. Encourage fluid intake after use.

- Stripping the membranes

This is a sterile procedure. Take caution not to rupture the membranes. Procedure releases prostaglandins.

- Amniotomy

Use only if committed to delivery. Check first through the membranes for presenting part, a loop of umbilical cord, or vasa previa (not always possible to feel). Note color of fluid. Evaluate for presence of cord and check FHR after amniotomy.

- Synthetic hygropic dilators
- Prostaglandins*

Prostaglandin E_2 gel 2.5 mL (0.5 mg prostaglandin) endocervically. May repeat q 6 hr three times

Dinoprostone (Cervidil) 10 mg vaginal insert applied in the posterior fornix. Remove with labor onset or after 12 hr.

Misoprostol (Cytotec) 25–50 μg inserted into the posterior fornix q 4 hr for up to 24 hr.

- Oxytocin*

A synthetic posterior pituitary hormone (pitocin, syntocinon, oxytocin), which is administered IV by controlled infusion pump.

The dosage is quite varied, ranging from initiation at 0.5–2 mU/min, with incremental increases of 1–2 mU/min every 15–60 min, and a maximum of 20–40 mU/min.

Possible side effects, requiring the oxytocin infusion to be stopped:

- Uterine hyperstimulation
- Fetal distress or nonreassuring FHR pattern
- Water intoxication
- Symptoms of uterine rupture

It is important to know the oxytocin protocols at your practice site, as well as rules regarding presence of clinical personnel in labor and delivery or in the hospital at the time oxytocin is used.

Continuous EFM is usually recommended throughout the oxytocin induction or augmentation of labor.

*All medications used to ripen the cervix have contraindications to use and to repeat dosing. Clinicians should review product literature to be sure they are using the medication safely.

Notes

Vaginal Birth after Cesarean (VBAC)[3]

All women with previous lower uterine segment cesarean sections should be encouraged to labor rather than plan a repeat cesarean section.

Data Collection

Patient history
- Type of cesarean scar
- Indication for cesarean section
- Length of labor
- Gestational age at time of cesarean section

Abdominal examination
- Inspection of abdominal scar

Pelvic examination
- Clinical pelvimetry
- Inspection of cervix and introitus, if no previous births have been vaginal

Risk Factors for Uterine Rupture

Any incision that extends into the uterine muscle mass of the uterine corpus or fundus including

- Previous classical cesarean
- Previous cesarean before 28 weeks
- Previous myomectomy that entered the uterine cavity

Labor Management

Management is the same as for normal labor, including the use of oxytocin and epidural anesthesia.

Signs and Symptoms of Uterine Rupture
- Abrupt change or cessation of uterine contractions
- Vaginal bleeding
- Loss of fetal station
- Abrupt change in the FHR

Other Considerations
- Documentation of previous incision type is necessary.

- There is an increased incidence of implantation of the placenta over the previous incision with the potential for placenta accreta.
- Asymptomatic scar dehiscence will heal by 6 weeks postpartum without any repair.

Preterm Labor[4]

Preterm, or premature, labor is labor commencing any time after the start of the twentieth week of gestation up to completion of the thirty-seventh week of gestation.

Signs and symptoms

- Painful menstrual-like cramps—may be confused with round ligament pain
- Dull low backache—different from the usual low backache a pregnant woman may have
- Suprapubic pain or pressure—may be confused with UTI
- Sensation of pelvic pressure or heaviness
- Change in character or amount of vaginal discharge (thicker, thinner, watery, bloody, brown, colorless)
- Diarrhea
- Unpalpated uterine contractions (painful or painless) felt more often than every 10 min for 1 hr or more and not relieved by lying down
- Premature rupture of the membranes

The signs and symptoms of preterm labor should be included as a routine part of the woman's prenatal education around 20 to 24 weeks gestation.

Management of Care

The midwife should provide the following care to a woman with a history of one previous preterm labor or birth and no signs and symptoms of preterm labor in this gestation:

- Monthly screening for asymptomatic bacteriuria
- Treatment of any vaginal and cervical infections
- Diet history and appropriate nutritional counseling
- Reinforcement of routine instructions about the signs and symptoms of preterm labor
- Counseling, if necessary, regarding cigarette, drug, and alcohol use
- Encouragement to communicate if she is having personal stress, so she can obtain appropriate help with stress reduction

If a woman has a history of two or more previous premature labors or births or has a multiple gestation and shows no signs and symptoms of preterm labor, then in addition to the above the midwife should do the following:

1. Conduct a vaginal examination every 2 weeks starting at 24 weeks gestation for cervical changes in position, consistency, effacement, and dilatation and for station of the presenting part. Research findings are inconsistent as to the predictive value of serial cervical examinations.

2. Recommend a change and/or reduction in workload if the woman's job involves heavy lifting, pushing or pulling, long hours, rotating shifts, or a lengthy commute.

3. Recommend use of condoms during sexual intercourse to prevent sexually transmitted diseases that might predispose the woman to premature rupture of the membranes and to prevent prostaglandin in the semen from causing uterine irritability.

4. Advise the woman to avoid nipple/breast stimulation to prevent uterine contractions.

Research has not shown that bed rest, home uterine activity monitoring (except for daily contact with a nurse), prophylactic oral tocolytic therapy, or prophylactic cerclage is effective in the prevention of preterm labor.

A woman with signs and symptoms of preterm labor, with or without any predisposing factors, should be seen immediately. You should notify your consulting physician and make the following assessment:

- History
  Signs and symptoms of preterm labor
  Signs and symptoms of UTI
  Signs and symptoms of vaginitis/cervicitis/sexually transmitted diseases
  Signs and symptoms of viral or bacterial infection
  Signs and symptoms of premature rupture of membranes
- Physical examination
  Vital signs (especially temperature and pulse)
  Evaluation of gestational age
  Evaluation of contractions*
  Evaluation of fetal heart rate*
  Abdominal palpation for presentation, position, multiple gestation, estimated fetal weight, and assessment of abdominal pain
  Costovertebral angle tenderness
  Assessment of low back pain and suprapubic pain
- Pelvic examination
  Speculum examination for evaluation of any existing vaginitis or cervicitis, sexually transmitted diseases, premature rupture of the membranes, bloody show, meconium
  Digital examination for evaluation of any existing cervical changes and of the station of the presenting part (a digital examination is not done if premature rupture of membranes is diagnosed on speculum examination)

- Laboratory tests
  STAT microscopic urinalysis
  Urine culture and sensitivity
  Wet mount of any vaginal discharge
  Cultures for group B streptococcus, gonorrhea, chlamydia, and any genital lesions
  CBC and differential (if the woman has signs and symptoms of infection)
  Fern test
  Nitrazine test

An accurate diagnosis of preterm labor is critical to determining the appropriate treatment. Contractions alone are not enough to diagnose preterm labor. A diagnosis of preterm labor is made between 20 and 37 weeks gestation when the woman is having uterine contractions (frequency of 5 to 8 min apart or four contractions in 20 min or eight in 60 min) *and* she exhibits (1) ruptured membranes *or* (2) intact membranes *and* (a) progressive cervical change, *or* (b) 2 cm dilatation, *or* (c) 80% effacement.

*How evaluation of the contractions and FHR is done may vary from place to place by institutional policy.

If the woman does not meet criteria for the diagnosis of preterm labor, she is sent home with the following instructions:

- Limit activity—curtail working hours in a nonstrenuous and nonstressful job or take a leave of absence from a strenuous or stressful job; do no heavy housework.
- Arrange for someone to help with household and child care responsibilities.
- Engage in no sexual activity until reevaluation in 1 week. Resumption of sexual activity depends on uterine activity and the presence of any predispos-

ing factors to preterm labor. If sexual activity is subsequently resumed, use condoms. If resumption of sexual activity causes an increase or recurrence of uterine contractions, the couple should be advised to abstain from sexual intercourse or other sexual activity that leads to orgasm in the woman.

- Return for routine prenatal care and reevaluation for preterm labor in 1 week.
- Continue to follow previous instructions on nutrition, recognizing signs and symptoms of preterm labor, stress reduction, and use of cigarettes, drugs, and alcohol.

Indications for Tocolysis
- Preterm labor before 34 weeks gestation
- Dilatation ≤ 4 cm

Contraindications for Tocolysis
- Fetal maturity
- Cervical dilatation of ≥ 5 cm
- Severe IUGR
- Fetal death or fetal anomaly incompatible with life
- Acute fetal distress
- Severe abruptio placenta
- Maternal hemodynamic instability (severe bleeding from any cause)
- Severe preeclampsia or eclampsia
- Chorioamnionitis

Contraindications to Specific Tocolytic Agents
Beta-adrenergic agonists (ritodrine and terbutaline)
- Poorly controlled diabetes
- Poorly controlled thyrotoxicosis
- Poorly controlled hypertension

Magnesium sulfate
- Renal failure
- Hypocalcemia
- Myasthenia gravis

Indomethacin

- Asthma
- Coronary artery disease
- Current or past gastrointestinal bleeding
- Renal failure
- Oligohydramnios
- Suspected fetal cardiac or renal anomaly

Nifedipine

- Maternal liver disease

Risk/benefit ratios must be considered with the use of tocolytics. Antenatal corticosteroid therapy has been shown to reduce the incidence and severity of respiratory distress syndrome, intraventricular hemorrhage, and neonatal mortality when administered between 24 and 34 weeks gestation to women at risk for preterm birth within 7 days. Optimal benefits begin 24 hr after initiation of therapy and last 7 days. It may be determined that the 24 hr needed for optimal benefit from the administration of corticosteroids is worth attempting at least 24 hr of tocolysis. Clearly, longer periods may be beneficial for very preterm infants.

Women receiving tocolytics for preterm labor require intensive support to help them overcome the physical side effects of the drugs. Continuous monitoring and support by the midwife to help alleviate the anxiety produced by these side effects contributes to the success of the tocolysis.

The follow-up for women whose preterm labor is stopped is weekly prenatal visits and vaginal examinations, preferably by the same examiner, to evaluate her for any cervical change. She should abstain from sexual intercourse or other sexual activity that leads to orgasm and continue to follow all previous instructions regarding work; nutrition; signs and symptoms of preterm labor; stress reduction; use of cigarettes, drugs, and alcohol; and household and child care responsibilities.

Midwifery management of progressive preterm labor is conducted in collaboration with the consulting physician. Every decision should have the goal of avoiding fetal asphyxia and trauma.

1. Route of delivery. Based on the fetal presentation and gestational age.
2. Type of analgesia and anesthesia. Narcotics, ataractics, and sedatives should not be used prior to delivery. Pudendal block or local infiltration should be used for episiotomy and repair; or, *if necessary*, a woman can have an epidural for comfort and control. Maternal hypotension from epidural anesthesia can be lessened by adequate preloading with crystalloid intravenous fluids.
3. Monitoring the fetus. A preterm baby has less reserve with which to tolerate the stresses of labor. Careful monitoring is also necessary for picking up tachycardia as a sign of intrauterine infection, especially if the membranes are ruptured.
4. Carefully weighing the usefulness of internal electronic fetal monitoring against the dangers involved in the application of the scalp clip. The preterm fetus has wider fontanels and a different skull bone density and consistency than a term fetus. The decision to use internal fetal monitoring must be based on a real need for internal electronic fetal monitoring and on gestational age.
5. Deciding whether an episiotomy is needed. The need for an episiotomy depends on the estimated fetal weight and the relaxation of the woman's perineum.
6. Arranging for the pediatrician/neonatologist to be notified and present for the delivery.

7. Making provisions for keeping the baby warm and for transporting the baby if necessary if the delivery did not take place in a Level III hospital. Neonatal mortality is reduced if delivery takes place in a tertiary hospital. If at all possible, it is better to transport the mother prior to delivery if this can be done safely.

Premature Rupture of the Membranes

Risk Factors

Incompetent cervix
Polyhydramnios
Fetal malpresentation
Multiple gestation
Vaginal/cervical infection

Complications Related to PROM

Preterm labor or birth
Chorioamnionitis
Umbilical cord compression

Data Base for Diagnosis

History—amount of fluid loss, inability to control flow with Kegel exercises, time of ROM, color of fluid, odor of fluid, last vaginal intercourse
Physical—abdominal assessment of decreased fluid
Pelvic—Sterile speculum examination for visible fluid on the perineum, in the vagina, at the cervix, or pooling in the vault; presence of vernix or lanugo; fluid expelled with Valsalva's maneuver
Laboratory tests—fern test, nitrazine response to alkaline amniotic fluid
Ultrasound—for oligohydramnios, if all of the above are negative and PROM is still suspected

Management

• Cultures—for group B strep (GBS), STDs, at the time of sterile speculum exam. Also evaluate for bacterial vaginosis.

- If ≤ 37 wks, GBS prophylaxis with IV antibiotics regardless of culture results
- Options
  1. Induction to effect delivery within 24 hours, based on concern that infections are more common with PROM
  2. Expectant management, based on understanding that 80% to 85% of term pregnancies begin labor within 24 hr of rupture, while observing closely for chorioamnionitis

During labor

- Assess temperature and pulse every 1–2 hr
- Monitor the fetal heart
- Avoid unnecessary examinations
- When pelvic examination is done, evaluate for increased vaginal temperature, odor, and color of fluid or discharge
- Note hydration carefully; dehydration is associated with elevated temperature

If expectant management is chosen
for women at term

- Management at home is acceptable for women with no other risk factors, who can take their own temperature, understand and manage the restrictions for pelvic rest, have telephone and transportation access, and have adequate support. Monitoring for chorioamnionitis is imperative.
- Check maternal temperature and pulse every 4 hr, uterine tenderness daily.
- Daily WBC count with differential.
- If the woman is hospitalized, check fetal heart tones every 4 hr.
- Evaluate fetal well-being with daily FMC, twice weekly NST and AFI, and weekly BPP.

Amnionitis and Chorioamnionitis

Signs and Symptoms

Maternal fever
Maternal tachycardia
Fetal tachycardia
Tender uterus
Elevation of vaginal temperature (warm to touch)
Foul-smelling amniotic fluid
Elevated WBC

Management

1. Facilitate delivery within 24 hr of diagnosis
2. Oxytocin induction or augmentation as needed to shorten labor
3. Rupture of forewaters if present
4. Internal electronic fetal monitoring
5. IV hydration with D_5RL
6. Vital signs hourly
7. Cesarean section is reserved for failure to progress to vaginal delivery or for worsening maternal or fetal condition
8. Consider antibiotic therapy, such as intravenous penicillin G, if delivery is not imminent
9. Notify pediatrics for the birth

Notes

Fetal Heart Rate Changes and Patterns[5]

Tachycardia

Tachycardia is a FHR of > 160 bpm for 10 min or more; frequently associated with decreased variability.

Causes

- Prematurity: < 28 wk gestation
- Maternal fever
- Fetal hypoxia—associated with a rising FHR base-line; may be an early indicator of fetal stress; if increase is persistent, fetal distress
- Maternal medications (e.g., terbutaline, ritodrine, theophylline, hydralazine, atenolol)
- Fetal cardiac anomaly
- Maternal dehydration
- Diabetic ketoacidosis
- Fetal anemia (Rh isoimmunization; feto-maternal bleed; abruptio placentae)
- Material hyperthyroidism

Management

- In a term fetus, tachycardia alone is not usually associated with a poor outcome
- A preterm or postterm fetus with uteroplacental insufficiency may be in distress
- Tachycardia with late decelerations or prolonged variable decelerations, with or without meconium, and absent variability is fetal distress

Bradycardia

Bradycardia is a baseline FHR of 100–119 bpm.
Marked bradycardia is a baseline FHR of < 100 bpm for > 10 min.

Causes

- Maternal hypothermia
- Fetal cord compression (prolapsed cord, complete or intermittent cord compression)

- Fetal hypoxia or asphyxia—usually preceded by nonreassuring FHR patterns and decreased variability
- Vagal stimulation (maternal Valsalva, vaginal examination, rapid descent, posterior/transverse position of fetal head)
- Fetal cardiac anomalies
- Maternal medications (e.g., propranolol, local anesthetics)

Management
- Assess for additional signs of fetal distress
- Check for prolapsed cord
- Assess duration of bradycardia
- Assess variability
- Assess for late or prolonged decelerations
- Ascertain expected length of time to delivery
- Change maternal position, if indicated
- Administer O_2 to mother, if indicated
- Consult, if indicated

Minimal or Absent Variability
(see also Fig. 11-5, p. 225)
- With internal fetal monitoring, variability is the most significant way to evaluate neurologic status and normal cardiac response
- Short-term variability can be assessed most accurately with an internal fetal scalp electrode
- Long-term variability can be assessed with the newer generation of Doppler equipment
- Average variability indicates that the autonomic nervous system, which controls the FHR, is mature and well-oxygenated
- Diminished variability (minimal or absent) or increased variability (marked) indicates depression of the autonomic nervous system

- Marked variability may be an early sign of mild hypoxia, but is usually associated with a normal pH

Causes
- Prematurity: < 28 wk gestation
- Drugs (e.g., analgesics/narcotics; barbiturates, tranquilizers, promethazine (Phenergan), ritodrine, terbutaline, anesthetics)
- Congenital/neurological anomalies (e.g., anencephaly)
- Fetal sleep cycles (should persist no longer than 80 min in the average fetus)
- Fetal hypoxia/acidosis (the most ominous explanation)

Management
- Identify cause and correct if possible
- If fetal hypoxia cannot be ruled out
    Stimulate fetal scalp (manual or vibroacoustic) with simultaneous continuous auscultation by Doppler monitoring (FHR acceleration even in the face of decelerations is associated with a pH > 7.25)
    Consider an internal fetal scalp electrode to determine the presence or absence of short-term variability and decelerations
    Assess hydration; start or increase IV hydration with a solution that does not contain glucose
    Administer oxygen by well-fitting face mask at 6–8 L/min
    Ascertain expected length of time to delivery
    Obtain maternal urine drug screen
    If accompanied by nonreassuring FHR deceleration patterns, tachycardia, and meconium, prepare the woman for expeditious delivery

Acceleration Patterns

- Periodic increases of the fetal heart rate above the baseline
- Reassuring indicator of fetal well-being—associated with a normal pH

Causes

- Fetal scalp stimulation
- Acoustic stimulation
- Fetal movement
- Vaginal examination
- Partial umbilical cord compression (observed more commonly with variable decelerations and breech presentations)

Deceleration Patterns

- Periodic FHR changes associated with uterine contractions
- Three patterns: early, late, variable

Early deceleration

- Caused by head compression
- Associated with cervical dilatation of 4 to 7 cm (pressure against the posterior fontanel)
- May return shortly before delivery (pressure from the perineal floor)

    Characteristics of early deceleration

- Reflects the shape of the uterine contraction pattern (usually uniform in shape)
- Onset corresponds with the onset of the related uterine contraction
- Total period of deceleration usually < 90 sec
- Deceleration ends when contraction ends
- Occurs with each contraction with only slight variation in the pattern from contraction to contraction

- Baseline usually within normal range (120–160 bpm)
- Deceleration usually not lower than 100 bpm at its lowest level

  MANAGEMENT
- Carefully differentiate from late deceleration pattern
- Does not require treatment or intervention

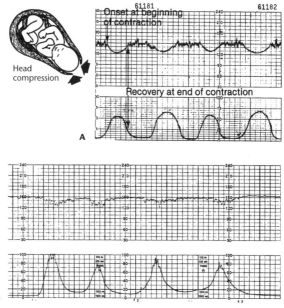

FIGURE 12-1   Early Deceleration.
A. Illustration with key points identified. Note the uniform shape that reflects the uterine contraction. B. Actual tracing.[6]

Source: Reproduced by permission from S. M. Tucker. *Pocket Guide to Fetal Monitoring,* 3d ed. St. Louis: Mosby Year Book, 1996.

Late deceleration
- Caused by uteroplacental insufficiency
- Uncorrected uteroplacental insufficiency is life-threatening; requires intervention to correct or expeditious delivery

CHARACTERISTICS
- Reflects shape of uterine contraction pattern (uniform in shape)
- Onset occurs late during the related uterine contraction (usually near peak of the contraction)
- Total period of deceleration usually < 90 sec
- Deceleration extends beyond end of contraction
- May or may not occur with each contraction
- Deceleration may be within normal range and as shallow as 10 bpm from the baseline FHR; or can extend beyond the normal FHR range (severity cannot be measured by depth of deceleration)

CAUSES OF CHRONIC AND ACUTE
UTEROPLACENTAL INSUFFICIENCY
- Fetal anemia (Rh sensitization, nonimmune hydrops, fetal-maternal hemorrhage)
- Maternal sickle cell crisis
- Intrauterine growth retardation associated with maternal chronic hypertension, lupus erythematosus, hyperthyroidism, intrauterine infection, poorly controlled diabetes
- Abnormal placentation (placenta previa, vasa previa, infarction of one or more lobes)
- Abruptio placenta associated with hypertension, cocaine use, overdistention of the uterus
- Hypertensive disorders (pregnancy-induced hypertension, chronic hypertension)
- Maternal hypotension syndrome (supine positioning, conduction anesthesia, severe dehydration, septic shock)

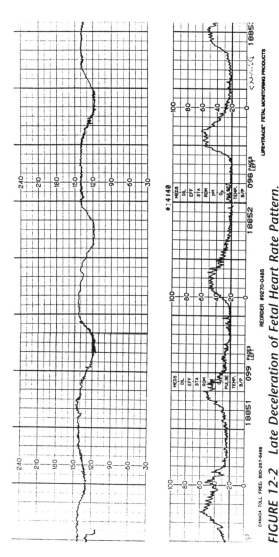

FIGURE 12-2 Late Deceleration of Fetal Heart Rate Pattern.
Baseline FHR 150 bpm. Note the onset of deceleration is near or after the peak of the contraction and returns to baseline after the contraction is over. Also note the minimal short term and long term variability, making this an ominous pattern reflecting uteroplacental insufficiency and fetal hypoxia.   *Source:* Tracing used with permission of C. Gegor, CNM.

- Hypertonic uterine contractions (use of oxytocin or prostaglandin E_2)
- Postmaturity

  MANAGEMENT

- Stop administration of oxytocin
- Hydrate with an intravenous solution that does not contain glucose
- Position woman on her left side with bed flat
- Administer oxygen at 6 to 8 L/min by well-fitting face mask
- Place internal fetal scalp electrode
- Perform scalp, acoustic, or manual stimulation of the fetus; if no response, obtain a fetal scalp pH
- Ascertain length of time to delivery
- Notify consulting physician
- If related to epidural anesthetic, check blood pressure, correct hypotension with hydration and/or ephedrine
- Explain seriousness to mother while preparing to expedite delivery
- Administer terbutaline, 0.25 mg SQ or 0.125 to 0.25 mg IV, if due to excessive uterine activity or when delays in operative intervention are unavoidable; tocolytic therapy should not be used to delay intervention

Variable deceleration caused by cord compression

  CAUSES OF CORD COMPRESSION

- Positioning of the cord around the neck and body
- True knots in the cord
- Frank and occult cord prolapse
- Decreased amniotic fluid
- Descent of breech through the pelvis in a breech presentation causing cord to be compressed between the baby's abdomen and the mother's pelvis

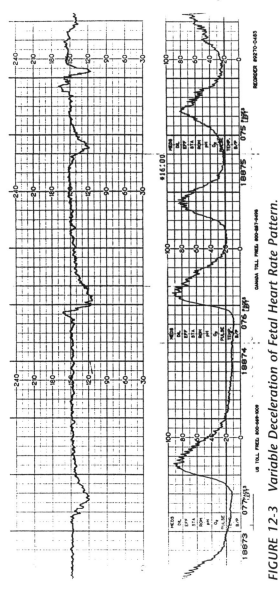

FIGURE 12-3 Variable Deceleration of Fetal Heart Rate Pattern.

Baseline FHR 140 bpm. Note the onset, return to baseline and shape of decelerations are in variable relationship to uterine contractions. Also note adequate long term and short term variability.

Source: Tracing used with permission of C. Gegor, CNM.

CHARACTERISTICS OF VARIABLE DECELERATION

- Shape of the FHR deceleration pattern does not reflect the shape of the uterine contractions
- Vary both in duration and in shape from occurrence to occurrence in relation to uterine contractions
- Onset is unpredictable and occurs at different times in relation to the onset and duration of the contractions
- Total period of deceleration varies from a few seconds to minutes
- In the well-oxygenated fetus, "shoulders," or small accelerations, may immediately precede the deceleration and may recur as the deceleration abruptly ends; these shoulders are reassuring and can be distinguished from their more ominous counterpart ("overshoot") because of the persistence of variability throughout the acceleration
- The baseline FHR is usually in the low normal or normal range
- The FHR usually decreases to below 100 bpm and can be as low as 50 to 60 bpm or lower
- Asystole, or junctional rhythm, of the FHR (30 bpm) may occur during the lowest point in the deceleration; repetition of this pattern may indicate that delivery is imminent
- Overshoot is a blunt acceleration occurring at the end of a variable deceleration with an absence of variability and slow return to baseline

MANAGEMENT

- The seriousness of variable decelerations depends on their frequency, depth, rate of return, effect on baseline FHR, and variability
- Variable decelerations that quickly return to a normal baseline with average variability are not associated with hypoxemia and acidosis

- Variable decelerations that have a slow return to baseline, an increased baseline rate (tachycardia), or absence of variability, regardless of depth of fall, may indicate a seriously compromised fetus; notify the consulting physician
- If the fetus has variable decelerations, regardless of type and recovery

  Change mother's position

  Do a vaginal examination to rule out prolapsed cord; ascertain if there has been rapid descent of the head with pressure from an incompletely dilated cervix; and ascertain the length of time to delivery

  Evaluate hydration status; initiate IV fluids

  Administer oxygen at 6 to 8 L/min with a well-fitting face mask

  May perform amnioinfusion if prolapsed cord and late decelerations have been ruled out

  Observe for tachycardia and loss of variability

Prolonged Deceleration Pattern

- Decelerations lasting longer than 60 to 90 sec
- Usually isolated events

Causes

- Umbilical cord compression
- Profound uteroplacental insufficiency
- Hypotension related to supine positioning or epidural or spinal anesthesia
- Hypertonic or tetanic contractions
- Paracervical anesthesia causing direct fetal uptake of local anesthetic, maternal hypotension, or uterine hypertonus
- Drugs such as Dramamine, Demerol (meperidine) when combined with Phenergan (promethazine), and cocaine
- Maternal hypoxia with seizures or acute respiratory depression

- Pelvic examination
- Maternal Valsalva
- Rapid descent of the fetal head

Management
- Management depends on the cause, length of deceleration, and recovery of the fetus after the pattern
- Common to have recovery with a period of tachycardia, decreased variability, and occasionally late decelerations
- If the cause is alleviated, the fetus usually recovers spontaneously
- If the deceleration is followed by FHR reactivity (FHR accelerations associated with fetal movement), outcome is generally good
- Protracted decelerations may precede fetal death
- If prolonged deceleration recurs, notify the consulting physician and prepare to expedite birth

Sinusoidal Pattern
- An undulating, repetitive, uniform FHR equally distributed 5 to 15 bpm above and below the baseline for at least 10 min
- An ominous pattern in the presence of chronic fetal anemia and severe hypoxia with acidosis

Characteristics
- The undulation has no relationship to either the contraction pattern or fetal movement
- Occurs at a rate of 2 to 6 cycles per min
- Absence of short-term variability
- No FHR accelerations after its occurrence

Causes
- Chronic fetal anemia (isoimmunization; abruptio placentae)
- Severe hypoxia with acidosis
- A benign form of sinusoidal pattern may follow the administration of drugs such as Stadol (butor-

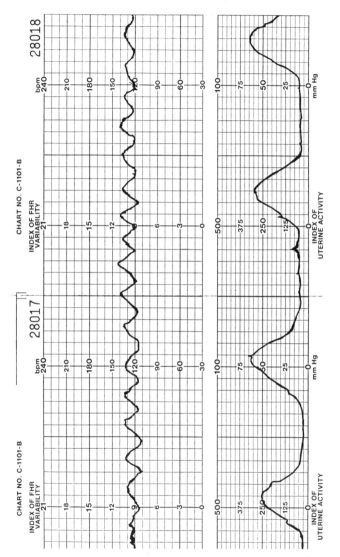

FIGURE 12-4   Sinusoidal Fetal Heart Rate Pattern.[7]
Source: Courtesy of Nancy McCluggage, CNM, MA.

phanol) or Demerol (meperidine); if acidosis or
anemia is not present, precipitation of this pattern
by administering analgesics has no significance

Management
- Immediate intervention to prevent fetal death
- Notify the consulting physician
- Prepare woman for cesarean birth
- Notify neonatal team to prepare for a potentially
  severely anemic, hypoxic, or acidotic newborn

Fetal Distress

Fetal stress: a situation in which the fetus is inter-
mittently experiencing hypoxemia; if transient, previously healthy fetuses are well equipped to tolerate these brief episodes without long-term sequelae

Fetal distress: a situation in which hypoxemia has
progressed to the extent that the fetus is now
hypoxic and acidotic (the fetus is experiencing
asphyxia: hypoxia with metabolic acidosis); this
may be a chronic condition usually secondary to
uteroplacental insufficiency, starting at some point
during the antepartal period or an acute condition
occurring during labor, or a combination of both.

*Causes of chronic fetal stress due
to uteroplacental insufficiency*
- Intrauterine growth retardation
- Chronic hypertension
- Maternal lupus erythematosus
- Cytomegalovirus
- Multiple gestation
- Abnormal placentation
- Postmaturity syndrome

Causes of acute fetal distress
- Onset of labor contractions when there has been
  chronic antepartal fetal stress: late decelerations
  and, less often, prolonged decelerations

- Compression of the umbilical cord (occult or obvious cord prolapse, nuchal cord, true knot, decreased amniotic fluid): variable decelerations and, less often, prolonged decelerations
- Rapid descent of the fetal head through the pelvis and breech deliveries: variable decelerations

Management

Meconium-stained amniotic fluid in the absence of other clinical signs of distress is not a sign of fetal distress; the presence of meconium with any sign of acute fetal distress, such as persistent late decelerations, variable decelerations, loss of variability and tachycardia, or sinusoidal pattern, is a serious indicator of fetal distress that requires prompt action.

- Notify the consulting physician
- Hydrate with an intravenous solution that does not contain glucose
- Discontinue any oxytocin stimulation
- Position the woman on her side
- Administer oxygen at 6 to 8 L/min with a well-fitting face mask
- Perform scalp, acoustic, or abdominal stimulation of the fetus; if no acceleration occurs in response, may obtain a fetal scalp blood sample for pH
- Administer tocolytic therapy with terbutaline 0.25 mg SQ or 0.125 to 0.25 mg IV, if:
  Fetal distress is related to uterine hyperstimulation
  There will be an unavoidable delay to operative intervention
- Perform amnioinfusion if there is cord compression
- If acute fetal distress is progressively worsening or is severe, initiate preparations for delivery by cesarean section

Cephalopelvic Disproportion (CPD)[8]

Disproportion between the size of the fetus and the size of the pelvis, in which a particular pelvis is not large enough to accommodate passage of a particular fetus to give birth vaginally. CPD may be evidenced by dysfunctional labor, a poorly flexed head, or an arrest of internal rotation and descent and may or may not be accompanied with caput and molding.

Indications

Indications that CPD may be present include the following.

- Excessively large fetus
- Woman's general body type
  - Shoulders wider than hips
  - Short, square stature
  - Short, broad hands and feet
  - Small shoe size
- History of pelvic fracture
- Spinal deformity, e.g., scoliosis or kyphosis
- Unilateral or bilateral marked lameness (lordosis)
- Orthopedic deformities, e.g., rickets, pinned hip
- Dysfunctional labor, uterine dysfunction
- Malpresentation or malposition

Evaluation

All women with an arrest of labor should be evaluated for CPD.

- Abdominal palpation for fetal lie, presentation, position, flexion, engagement, and station; estimated fetal weight
- Assessment of uterine contractions for frequency, duration, intensity, and changes from earlier labor; dysfunctional labor is commonly seen in CPD
- Pelvic examination to determine position of presenting part, engagement, station, degree of flexion, synclitism/asynclitism, formation of caput,

molding, progress (or lack) of dilatation and effacement, and descent
- Clinical pelvimetry

Management

Management of suspected CPD may include some of the following:

- Maternal position changes
- Artificial rupture of membranes
- Ambulation of the mother
- Rest and hydration of the mother, if exhaustion is present
- Oxytocin to increase uterine contractions
- Administration of an epidural for maternal rest and relaxation
- Manual rotation of the fetal head to alter the position of the head

Suspected CPD

Management of suspected CPD and uterine dysfunction must be managed in a timely fashion with physician consultation due to these possible related outcomes:

- Fetal damage
- Fetal or neonatal death
- Intrauterine infection
- Uterine rupture
- Maternal death

If the measures listed for management of CPD are unsuccessful, intervention, including cesarean section, is indicated.

Deep Transverse Arrest[9]

Deep transverse arrest is associated with platypelloid and android pelvic types, which inhibit the mechanism of labor of internal rotation to bring the sagittal suture from being in the transverse diameter to being in the anteroposterior diameter of the mother's pelvis.

Deep transverse arrest should be considered when there is:

- Prolonged second-stage labor
- Fetal sagittal suture in transverse diameter of maternal pelvis
- Second-stage hypotonic uterine dysfunction
- Excessive molding of the fetal head
- Formation of considerable caput succedaneum

Means to avoid deep transverse arrest when potential is suspected

- Assume positions to promote pushing, such as squatting or kneeling
- Keep mother well-hydrated in the second stage
- Avoid exhaustion: push only with peak of contraction or when strong urge to push

Management of Deep Transverse Arrest
- Careful monitoring of progress
- Determine engagement with Leopold's fourth maneuver
- Improve uterine activity with oxytocin
- Correct maternal exhaustion

Suspected CPD should be discussed with the consulting physician. When management efforts do not facilitate delivery, the consultant physician must evaluate for use of forceps, vacuum extraction, or cesarean section.

Uterine Dysfunction[10]
Uterine dysfunction is identified as prolongation of any phase or stage of labor typified by a lack of progress of cervical dilatation or descent of the presenting part. Intensity of contractions may be measured by abdominal palpation and cervical examination to determine progress. An intrauterine pressure catheter (IUPC) may also be useful to determine intensity of contractions.

Hypotonic Uterine Contractions

Contractions are not painful, but have a normal gradient pattern (greatest intensity in fundus, weakest in cervix), poor tone or intensity, and are inadequate to cause progressive dilatation. The labor will have progressed normally into the active phase or to second stage, then diminished.

Assess
- Frequency, duration and intensity of contractions; any changes
- Maternal exhaustion
- Fetal well-being
- Maternal environment for stress factors
- Presentation, position, engagement, and station
- For CPD, caput, flexion, asynclitism, pelvic adequacy
- Progress of labor: effacement, dilatation, descent
- Membranes intact/ruptured? fluid clear? ruptured how long?
- Maternal vital signs

Management options
In collaboration with the consulting physician

- Modify stress in environment
- Correct maternal exhaustion
- Administer epidural anesthesia for pain relief or release from tension or fear
- Facilitate ambulation, shower, tub, Jacuzzi
- Give enema
- Rupture membranes
- Stimulate nipples
- Stimulation with oxytocin

Hypertonic Uterine Contractions

Contractions with a distorted pressure gradient (midportion of uterus more contractile than fundus and overall hypertonicity), which may lead to maternal exhaustion and fetal intolerance of labor. Occurs early in labor during latent phase.

Assess
- Usually in primigravidas
- Pain of contractions often greater than intensity of contractions
- Frequency, length, and intensity of contractions
- Progress of cervical effacement and dilatation

Management
In collaboration with the consulting physician, stop the discoordinated contraction pattern with induced rest with a combination of morphine and a barbituate

Maternal Exhaustion (Maternal Distress: Ketoacidosis)[11]

Signs and Symptoms

History
- Weakness, apathy, anxiety
- Prolonged labor
- Dehydration (dry lips and mouth, parched throat)

Physical
- Restlessness
- Rising pulse
- Elevated temperature
- Circumoral pallor
- Vomiting

Laboratory
- Concentrated urine (elevated specific gravity)
- Urine ketones

Management
- Prevention is best
- Correction of fluid/electrolyte imbalance
- Consultation regarding abnormal length of phases of labor

Uterine Rupture[12]

Most Common Causes

- Previous surgery to the fundus or corpus of the uterus
- Injudicious use of oxytocin induction or augmentation of labor
- Abnormal presentations (especially in the thinned-out lower uterine segment of a grand multipara)

Signs and Symptoms

These may be dramatic or quiet.

Dramatic

- Sharp, shooting pain in lower abdomen at height of a severe contraction
- Cessation of uterine contractions with great relief from previous pain
- Vaginal bleeding (slight amount or hemorrhage)
- Signs and symptoms of shock: elevated pulse (rapid and thready); decreased blood pressure; pallor; cold, clammy skin; apprehensiveness or feeling of impending doom or death; air hunger (shortness of breath); restlessness; and visual disturbances
- Findings on abdominal palpation are changed from previous findings
  - Presenting part is now movable above the pelvic inlet
  - May be dramatic repositioning or relocation of the fetus in the mother's abdomen
  - Fetal parts are more easily palpated
  - Fetal movements may become violent and then decrease to no fetal movements and no fetal heart tones (FHT), or there may be continuing FHT
  - Round, firm (contracted) uterus is felt beside the fetus (fetus is felt outside of the uterus)

Quiet (silent)

- Possible vomiting
- Increased tenderness over the abdomen
- Severe suprapubic pain
- Hypotonic uterine contractions
- Lack of further progress in labor
- Feeling of faintness
- Hematuria (eventually)
- Vaginal bleeding (eventually)
- Some pain (eventually)
- Signs of progressive shock from blood loss with a rising and rapid pulse rate and pallor (eventually)
- Contractions may continue with no effect on the cervix; or no contractions may be felt
- FHT may be lost

Management

- Immediately have consulting physician, anesthesia, and operating room staff notified.
- Start two intravenous infusion routes with 16-gauge intracatheters: one for electrolyte solutions (e.g., lactated Ringer's solution) and the other for the blood transfusion (keep the infusion line open with normal saline until the blood is obtained).
- Notify the blood bank of your need for a STAT blood transfusion. Estimate the number of units needed as well as the probable need for fresh frozen plasma.
- Administer oxygen.
- Make all preparations for immediate abdominal surgery (laparotomy and hysterectomy).
- In desperate situations institute aortic compression and add oxytocin to the IV solution.

Blood Transfusion Reactions[13]

Signs and Symptoms

Subjective

Lumbar/leg pain

Feeling of fullness in the head

Vertigo

Headache

Chest constriction

Feeling cold

Vague muscle weakness, extending from the extremities to the trunk

Nausea

Apprehensiveness

Muscle cramps

Paresthesia of hands, fingers, feet, tongue and perioral area

Objective

Fever

Chills

Shortness of breath

Tachycardia

Hypotension

Decreased urine output

Urticaria

Edema

Diarrhea

Slow, irregular pulse

Convulsions

Rales, respiratory stridor

Spasms of the hands and feet

Hyperactive reflexes

Neck vein distention

Cyanosis

Management
- Stop the transfusion.
- Flush the IV tubing and keep the IV route open with normal saline.
- Notify the consulting physician of the reaction so the physician can determine which complication has occurred and its management.
- Notify the blood bank and save the unit of blood that caused the reaction for further analysis.

Notes

Umbilical Cord Prolapse[14]

Precipitating Causes

1. An unengaged head, breech presentation, compound presentation, transverse lie, small fetus (less than 2000 grams or whose presenting part does not fill the pelvis), or second-born twin and
   a. Ruptured membranes
   b. Administration of an enema if the membranes are ruptured
   c. Amniotomy
   d. Vaginal examination causing rupture of the membranes in the presence of tense, bulging membranes
   e. Spontaneous rupture of the membranes
2. Displacement of the vertex during fetal assessment or obstetric manipulation (e.g., manual rotation of the head; placement of forceps other than outlet forceps)

Any time the membranes rupture, your first action should be to check the fetal heart and then to perform a vaginal examination to feel for a prolapsed cord. The following actions are taken in the presence of a prolapsed cord

1. Place your entire hand into the woman's vagina and hold the presenting part up off the umbilical cord at the pelvic inlet.
2. Do not under any circumstances attempt to replace the cord—manipulation may cause cord spasm causing further cord compression.
3. Inform the woman of what has happened and elicit her cooperation.
4. Summon help. Warn the woman and, if necessary, yell to get attention.
5. Have someone give the physician a STAT call.

6. Direct others to get the woman into knee-chest or Trendelenburg position.

7. If the cord is protruding from the vagina, direct others to wrap it loosely with gauze soaked with warm normal saline.

8. Do not palpate for or rely on cord pulsations as an indicator of fetal life or well-being.

9. Monitor the FHT as continuously as possible with doppler, EFM, or ultrasound visualization of fetal heart movement.

10. Direct others to prepare for an emergency cesarean section.

11. Under no circumstances remove your hand from the woman's vagina or from the presenting part until the baby is delivered (probably by cesarean section).

12. May request an injection of 0.25 mg terbutaline, given subcutaneously, if the woman is contracting.

An alternative method can be used with an *unengaged* presenting part. This method is to insert a #16 Foley catheter, fill the bladder with 500 cc of sterile water or normal saline, and clamp the catheter while your hand is in the vagina displacing the fetal head off the umbilical cord. The full bladder then displaces the presenting part and alleviates the cord compression. This technique can also be used when the presenting part is engaged if the woman is a multipara. It will be necessary, however, for you to displace the presenting part out of the pelvis with your hand before filling the bladder. Pressure on the presenting part should be evenly distributed during this maneuver. Once the bladder is filled you should again check the woman vaginally to determine that the presenting part is indeed displaced. The fetal heart should be continually electronically monitored. If bradycardia recurs, reinsert your hand into the vagina to assure that the fetal head is off the cord.

Shoulder Dystocia[15]

Shoulder dystocia should be anticipated whenever you note any of the following findings or conditions

1. Maternal diabetes, particularly gestational or class A diabetes
2. Obstetric history of large babies
3. Family history of large siblings
4. Maternal obesity
5. Postdates
6. Large fetus, as determined by palpation or ultrasound diagnosis of macrosomia
7. Varney's predictive factor of an estimated fetal weight 1 lb or more greater than the woman's largest previous baby
8. Obstetric history of a difficult delivery
9. Cephalopelvic disproportion
10. Desultory active phase of the first stage of labor
11. Prolonged second stage of labor
12. Indication of the need for midpelvic rotation and/or delivery with either forceps or vacuum extractor. This is the predictive factor that most likely will be combined with a large fetus, prolonged second stage of labor, and cephalopelvic disproportion and that most strongly indicates consideration of a cesarean section.

Management of Shoulder Dystocia

The first six steps occur concurrently; the rest occur in sequence.

1. *Stay calm.* You know what to do and will effectively manage this situation.
2. *Request that your consulting physician be called immediately.*

3. *Request readiness for a full-scale newborn resuscitation effort.*

4. *Request readiness for an immediate postpartum hemorrhage.* Include a request for a straight catheter.

5. Briefly tell the mother that there is a problem with delivery of the baby's shoulders, that you and the baby need her cooperation, and that you will be doing things that will hurt her. Tell her that she must *not* push now.

6. *Place the woman in an exaggerated lithotomy position (McRoberts maneuver).*

7. *Check the position of the shoulders. Using your entire hands, rotate the shoulders into one of the oblique diameters of the pelvis* if they are in either the transverse or anteroposterior diameter of the mother's pelvis.

   Again, instruct the mother not to push. *Under no circumstances make the mistake of thinking that moving the head will move the shoulders. All you will do is twist the baby's neck; this may result in injury of the brachial or cervical nerve plexus or fracture of the cervical vertebrae.*

8. *Have someone else apply suprapubic pressure while you exert your usual downward and outward pressure on the side of the baby's head.* Excessive force or traction on the baby's head may result in nerve palsy. *Under no circumstances should you allow fundal pressure to be given.*

9. If the baby has not delivered, take the time (approximately 40 to 45 sec) to give yourself every piece of knowledge, advantage, and bit of room to deliver the shoulders:

   a. *Catheterize the woman to empty her bladder* if you don't know if she entered delivery with an empty bladder.

   b. *Ascertain the need to cut or enlarge the epi-siotomy.*
   c. *Do a vaginal examination to rule out other causes of labor dystocia after the head is born.* This requires the insertion of your entire examining hand as far as you can.
10. *If the labor dystocia is diagnosed as resulting from shoulder dystocia, attempt again to deliver the baby by again having someone apply suprapubic pressure* while you exert firm, but not excessive, downward and outward pressure on the side of the baby's head.
11. (Steps 11 and 12 are reversible.) *If the baby has not delivered, do the corkscrew maneuver, utilizing the screw principle of Woods.* Always rotate the body of the baby so that the back is rotated ante-riorly (back up).
12. *If the baby still has not delivered, deliver the posterior arm.* Resist any temptation to hook your fingers under the baby's axilla or into the armpit.
13. *Attempt to deliver the baby now by the combination of suprapubic pressure and downward and outward pressure on the side of the baby's head* (see Step 8).
14. *If the baby has not delivered, rotate the baby's body 180° again* (as in Step 11). This will substitute the now delivered posterior shoulder for the anterior shoulder.

   In an exceptionally rare situation (which the majority of midwives will not see in an entire career), the baby will not have delivered and you then proceed to the next step.
15. *Traditionally the next step was to break the baby's clavicle,* and for some it may still be the next step. The anterior clavicle is broken first in order to col-lapse the anterior shoulder and dislodge it from behind the symphysis pubis.

16. *For other practitioners the next step is to use the Zavanelli maneuver to replace the head back into the vagina followed by delivery of the baby by cesarean section.* To replace the head, reverse the mechanisms of labor and depress the posterior vaginal wall while supporting the head.

    The Zavanelli maneuver is a final option, unless you found an obstructive tumor on vaginal examination in Step 9c. In such a situation you would go directly to the Zavanelli maneuver, as it is not possible to deliver the baby vaginally.

Charting
Document

- Basis for diagnosis of shoulder dystocia
- Steps taken, in sequence and approximate amount of time for each
- All professionals involved
- Apparent outcomes

Delivery of the Infant with a Face Presentation

Many babies with face presentations begin labor either in a brow presentation or with a hyperextended head and convert to a face presentation during descent. The diagnosis of a face presentation is based on the following:

1. Abdominal palpation (Leopold's third and fourth maneuvers)—the occipital bone is prominent and easily palpable; the head may feel larger than anticipated compared with a well-flexed head.

2. Pelvic examination—you may be unable to identify both fontanels clearly or may feel only the anterior fontanel if the baby is in a hyperextended presentation. With a brow presentation, you will feel the brow and possibly the anterior fontanel, but no other common identifying landmarks. In a face presentation, you will be able to feel the baby's

eyes, nose, mouth, and chin, although initially the presenting part may feel soft and lumpy, similar to a breech presentation, rather than firm and smooth. On further examination and palpation, the landmarks of the face become evident. If the membranes are ruptured, the baby may even suck your finger as you approach the mouth.

Once you have diagnosed a face presentation, do not apply an internal electrode, as this device will damage the infant's face or may be inadvertently applied to an eyelid.

During internal rotation, the chin either rotates anteriorly or posteriorly.

Anteriorly:

> 45° for RMA and LMA to MA
> 90° for RMT and LMT to MA
> 135° for RMP and LMP to MA

Posteriorly:

> 45° for RMP and LMP to MP

If the chin rotates posteriorly into a mentum posterior position, the mechanisms of labor cease because the baby cannot deliver vaginally from this position. Delivery is by cesarean section.

Birth of the head in a mentum anterior position is by a double mechanism of extension followed by flexion. Extension is maintained until the chin is born by escaping beneath the symphysis pubis. The submental area beneath the chin impinges beneath the symphysis pubis and becomes the pivotal point for the delivery of the rest of the head by flexion. The rest of the head is born sequentially starting with the mouth, then the nose, eyes, brow, anterior fontanel, and posterior fontanel, and ending with the occiput as the head flexes.

Management of a Face Presentation

1. Recognize that the position is a face presentation and notify the consulting physician of this malpresentation.

2. Reevaluate the adequacy of the pelvis and consult with the physician if there is a question of possible CPD.

3. Closely monitor the mechanism of internal rotation. Immediately inform the physician if rotation is to a direct mentum posterior position.

4. For delivery of the head:

   a. Apply pressure on the fetal brow to maintain extension until the chin is born. This is done by pressing on the posterior end of the perineal body as the vulvovaginal orifice distends. Protect your gloved hand from contamination from the rectum during this maneuver by covering it with a towel.

   b. Control the head to allow the gradual flexion and birth of the remainder of the head. Most face presentations deliver spontaneously with little need for extensive hand maneuvers.

5. Request that the pediatrician/neonatal nurse practitioner attend the delivery. If there is extensive edema of the neck (trachea), nose, and mouth, respiratory function may be compromised.

6. Reassure parents, family, and significant others that the position of the head and neck of the baby (neck extended, head fallen backwards), the long molded head, and the extensive swelling of the features of the face normally noticeably improve in a day or two and completely disappear in a few days.

Delivery of Infants in Breech Presentations

Before the actual delivery begins, the following should have taken place

1. Complete cervical dilatation
2. Elimination of any question about the adequacy of the pelvis
3. Emptying of the bladder
4. Episiotomy cut if needed
5. Presence of an effective maternal pushing effort
6. Preparation for newborn resuscitation
7. Woman positioned so there is plenty of room for lateral flexion and downward traction in the lithotomy position either in stirrups or at the edge of a bed
8. Consulting physician notified and either present or immediately available

If this is an in-hospital emergency situation in which the midwife is delivering a woman she or he has not seen before and has not previously had time to examine, the midwife's first action should be to inform the attending nursing staff of the situation and request that in addition to a STAT call being placed for the physician, an anesthesiologist or nurse anesthetist and a pediatrician or neonatal clinical nurse specialist or practitioner should also be called to stand by in case they are needed.

The midwife facilitates the mechanisms of labor of a breech presentation, follows the principle of nonintervention as long as progress is visible, and does manual extraction manipulations as indicated. It helps to visualize the mechanisms of labor if you remember that they *are in sequence for birth of the buttocks, birth of the shoulders, and birth of the head,* in that order.

Correlation of Mechanisms of Labor and Hand Maneuvers for Delivery of a Breech Presentation[16]

1, 2, 3. Mechanism of labor
a. Descent occurs throughout.

b. Engagement of the hips takes place in an RSA position with the sacrum in the right anterior portion of the mother's pelvis and the bitrochanteric diameter in the right oblique diameter of the mother's pelvis.

c. Internal rotation of the buttocks 45° from RSA to RST. This brings the anterior hip, which descended more rapidly than the posterior hip and initiated internal rotation when it encountered resistance from the pelvic floor, 45° forward (anterior) to underneath the pubic arch. The bitrochanteric diameter is now in the anteroposterior diameter of the mother's pelvis.

1, 2, 3. Hand maneuvers

Normally you will not need to intervene in the first three mechanisms of labor. In the event that the breech does not descend, rule out cephalopelvic disproportion and hydrocephalus. It is possible, however, that failure to descend may be due to a splinting effect caused when it is a frank breech and the extension of the legs across the baby's abdomen prevents the fetus from maneuvering and arrests progress. The Pinard maneuver will enable you to bring down the feet and legs, changing the presentation to a footling breech. This is done as follows:

a. With your vaginal hand (left hand if the baby is in a left sacrum position, right hand if the baby is in a right sacrum position) follow the posterior side of a thigh up from the buttocks to the popliteal fossa behind the knee. Your thumb will be on the anterior side of the thigh.

b. Move the leg laterally away from the midline and the baby's body while pressing in the popliteal fossa. This will cause the leg to flex at the knee, thereby bringing the foot, which was at the level of the baby's face and out of reach, down to where you can grasp it.

c. Bring the leg down by drawing it across the baby's abdomen in its natural range of motion and down for its delivery.

d. Repeat for the other thigh, leg, and foot.

4. Mechanism of labor

Birth of the buttocks by lateral flexion. When born spontaneously, the posterior hip is born first; the anterior hip impinges beneath the symphysis pubis and serves as the pivoting point for the lateral flexion necessary for the posterior hip to follow the curve of Carus to birth. The baby's body then straightens out as the anterior hip is born.

The legs and feet usually follow the birth of the breech and are also born spontaneously.

4. Hand maneuvers

You should keep your hands off the baby. The one exception is if the baby is in a frank breech presentation and the extended legs prevent the necessary lateral flexion for birth of the buttocks. In such an event, the Pinard maneuver is used for delivery of the feet and legs and then the buttocks. Prior to using this maneuver (i.e., during descent), you must clearly rule out cephalopelvic disproportion.

5. Mechanism of labor

(a) External rotation of the buttocks 45° from RST to RSA and (b) engagement of the shoulders with the bisacromial diameter in the right oblique diameter of the mother's pelvis (the same as for engagement of the buttocks). These two mechanisms occur simultaneously, with the external rotation of the buttocks being visible evidence of the entry of the shoulders into the true pelvis as the body untwists and aligns itself with the descending shoulders. Descent of the shoulders after their engagement is rapid.

5. Hand maneuvers

Continue a hands-off approach.

a. There is no need to facilitate the progress of the mechanisms of labor until the baby is born up to the umbilicus. After that, the remainder of the baby needs to be born in 3 to 5 min to avoid anoxia.

b. Traction exerted on the baby prior to birth up to the umbilicus may cause (1) the arms to fly up in a reflex action, thereby extending them above, over, or behind the head and causing later difficulties in the delivery, and/or (2) the head to deflex, which may cause dangerous problems with birth of the head.

c. Natural progress using the bulk of the breech maintains cervical dilatation and lessens the possibility that the cervix may clamp around the baby's head or neck.

It is a good time to request a warm, dry towel to use next. When the baby is born up to the umbilicus you do two things:

a. Pull down a good-sized loop of umbilical cord to prevent stress on its insertion in the umbilicus during the rest of the delivery.

b. Place the warm towel around the baby from just below the umbilicus down. This helps keep the baby warm and gives you a nonslippery hold on the baby, which is essential both for safety and to allow you to exert the traction now needed.

6. Mechanism of labor

Internal rotation of the shoulders 45°, bringing the bisacromial diameter of the fetus from the right oblique diameter to the anteroposterior diameter of the mother's pelvis. This is evidenced externally when the delivered body also rotates and the sacrum returns to an RST position from an RSA position.

6. Hand maneuvers

After birth of the umbilicus, you exert downward and outward traction while facilitating internal rotation of the shoulders by rotating the body so the sacrum again rotates from RSA to RST. To do this safely without injury to internal organs or structures (e.g., kidneys, adrenal glands) resulting from the pressure you apply in order to exert traction, the placement of your hands on bone is vitally important.

a. Grasp the baby on its hips with your thumbs on either sacroiliac region and your fingers on the corresponding iliac crests.
b. Continue this traction until you can see not only the lower half of the scapula of the anterior shoulder but also its corresponding axilla.

7. Mechanism of labor

Birth of the shoulders by lateral flexion. When born spontaneously, the anterior shoulder impinges beneath the symphysis pubis and serves as the pivotal point for the lateral flexion necessary for delivery of the posterior shoulder via the curve of Carus. Birth of the anterior shoulder then follows as the body straightens out.

7. Hand maneuvers

It doesn't matter which shoulder is delivered first. The following methodology is in accord with the mechanisms of labor.

a. Grasp the feet of the baby in one hand with your index finger between the legs and your middle finger and thumb each encircling a leg.

b. Holding the baby by its feet, exert upward traction for the entire body and draw the baby's abdomen toward the mother's inner thigh. Be careful to keep the back from turning upwards so that the head will enter the pelvis in the transverse diameter.

c. This draws the posterior shoulder over the perineum to birth, followed by the arm and hand of the same side.

d. If necessary, such as when the arm has become extended, deliver the arm first, as follows:

   (1) Insert the fingers of your vaginal hand and follow the humerus of the posterior arm until you feel the elbow.

   (2) Use these fingers now as a splint for the arm and sweep it across the baby's chest downward to delivery.

e. Now exert downward traction on the baby for delivery of the anterior shoulder, arm, and hand. To exert this downward traction, again place your hands on the baby's hips as you did in Step 6.

f. Again, if necessary, such as when the arm has become extended, deliver the arm first, as described in Step 7d.

g. If there is a nuchal arm (the arm is extended from the shoulder but flexed at the elbow so that the lower arm is wedged behind the head), attempts to deliver it the same way as for extended arms as in Steps 7d and 7f will not work. Delivery of a nuchal arm is as follows:

   (1) Grasp the baby by placing your hands on the baby's hips as you did for Step 6.

   (2) Rotate the baby's body 90° to 180° in the direction in which the hand behind the head is

pointing until the arm is dislodged from behind the head. This is accomplished by the friction of the body rotating against the vaginal outlet in a direction that forces the elbow toward the face and places the arm in a position from which it can now be delivered.

(3) Deliver the arm as for an extended arm as described in Step 7d.

(4) If both arms are nuchal arms, then repeat this process for the other arm, rotating the baby in the direction indicated, after delivery of the first arm.

h. If all else fails, break the arm by hooking a finger over it and pulling on it. Such trauma is indicated when weighed against the baby's life. Such a fracture usually heals well without deformity.

8. Mechanism of labor

Engagement of the head takes place with the sagittal suture in either the transverse or left oblique diameter of the mother's pelvis and the occiput in the right side of the pelvis. The head enters the pelvis as the shoulders near the outlet and may engage prior to or after internal rotation of the shoulders—which explains why engagement is in either the transverse or oblique diameter of the pelvic inlet.

8. Hand maneuvers

Suprapubic pressure should be applied by an assistant to maintain the normal flexion of the baby's head. Suprapubic pressure is continued until the head is born.

9. Mechanism of labor

Internal rotation of the head 45° or 90°, bringing the sagittal suture from the left oblique or transverse diameter, respectively, into the anteroposterior diameter of the mother's pelvis with the occiput directly anterior and the brow in the hollow of the sacrum of the mother's pelvis. This rotation is evidenced externally because the delivered body also rotates, thereby bringing the bisacromial diameter of the shoulders into the horizontal plane of the mother and the sacrum into a direct anterior position (i.e., the back of the baby is upward and the baby is facing down).

9. Hand maneuvers

Facilitate rotation of the head to an occiput anterior position:

    a. Grasp the baby by placing your hands on the baby's hips as you did for Step 6.

    b. Monitor the rotation of the head by observing the external rotation of the body.

    c. Do not allow the head to rotate to an occiput posterior position as evidenced by rotation of the back posteriorly. If this should begin to occur, counteract by rotating the baby so its back is anterior. Rotation of the head posteriorly so that the occiput is posterior and the chin is facing the symphysis pubis makes delivery of the head extremely difficult and dangerous.

10. Mechanism of labor

Birth of the head by flexion.

10. Hand maneuvers

It is vital to keep the head flexed at this time by continuing suprapubic pressure and by using the Mauriceau-Smellie-Veit maneuver. This maneuver is performed as follows:

    a. One hand is introduced into the vagina palmar side up beneath the baby's face.

      (1) Place the index finger of this hand in the baby's mouth and press the back of the finger against the maxilla (upper jaw bone), i.e., against the roof of the mouth.

    (2) This finger is used to help keep the head in flexion and should *never* be used for traction.

    (3) Take care not to allow the finger to slip and apply pressure and/or traction against the mandible (lower jaw bone) and the base of the tongue, as this could cause serious injury.

    (4) Use the rest of this hand to support the body of the baby, which is positioned astride your arm.

b. Your other hand is placed on the baby's upper back with your index finger hooked over one shoulder on one side of the neck and your middle finger hooked over the other shoulder on the other side of the neck.

    (1) This hand will be used for exerting traction.

    (2) Place your hooking fingers as far as possible away from the neck to avoid pressure on the cervical or brachial nerve plexuses.

    (3) Grasp the shoulders with your thumb and remaining fingers.

c. Modifications of the Mauriceau-Smellie-Veit maneuver include the following:

    (1) Placement of the index and fourth fingers of the lower hand on the upper jaw (malar bones) on either side of the nose with the middle finger in the baby's mouth. Another alternative is to put the index and fourth finger on the infraorbital ridge and the middle finger in the mouth, but you must be *extremely* careful not to misplace your fingers and damage the baby's eyes. These modifications allow you to exert traction with your lower hand.

    (2) Extension of one or two fingers (index or index and middle fingers) of the upper hand up the back of the baby's neck under the symphysis pubis and up the occiput, thereby splinting the baby's neck, keeping the head from extending, and facilitating flexion.

d. Apply downward and outward traction with your hand on the baby's shoulders until you can see the suboccipital region (hair line) under the symphysis pubis.

e. Now apply upward traction while elevating the body of the baby so that the chin, mouth, nose, eyes, brow, anterior fontanel, posterior fontanel, and occiput follow the curve of Carus and are born in sequence as the head remains flexed for birth.

f. Birth of the head is controlled by the pressure of your hands. If this step proceeds too fast and the head pops out, intracranial damage may result; and if it is too slow, hypoxia becomes a concern.

Multiple Gestation
Early identification is essential to minimize complications of multiple pregnancy.

Signs and Symptoms
- Large for dates uterine size or fundal height
- Rapid growth of uterus in second trimester
- Family history of twins
- Use of infertility drugs
- Abdominal palpation of three or more large parts or multiple small parts, especially in third trimester
- Auscultation of more than one clearly distinct FHT

Diagnosis
- Clinical findings
- Ultrasound examination—multiple gestations can be identified as early as 6 to 7 wk and should absolutely be seen by 10 wk

Associated High-Risk Situations
- Preterm labor
- Preeclampsia
- IUGR/discordant growth
- Polyhydraminos

Antepartum Management
- Collaboration with physician consultant
- Increased nutritional intake, especially protein and calories
- Increased rest periods
- More frequent prenatal visits for close observation of fetal growth and symptoms of cervical change or preterm labor
- Increased psychosocial support
  - Physical discomforts more extreme
  - Distorted body image
  - Baby care preparations difficult
  - Increased financial stress
- Close evaluation of fetal growth
  - Serial ultrasound examinations from 28 weeks to term, every 3 to 4 wk
  - If both babies are well grown, continue to manage as normal fetuses
  - If one or both have discordant growth, should be managed as high-risk with physician consultation
- Initiate BPP and NST as indicated

Delivery of a Woman with Multiple Gestation[17]
The cardinal rules and essential steps for assisting the labor and delivery of a woman with multiple gestation are:

1. Analgesics and sedatives should not be used because the fetuses are often preterm or small for gestational age.
2. Woman has a patent IV.
3. Woman's bladder is empty at start of the delivery.
4. Physician is notified and present at the start of the delivery.
5. Anesthesia personnel are notified and on standby.
6. Pediatrician is notified and present.
7. Woman is in lithotomy position to allow plenty of room for manipulations.

8. Nursing personnel are alerted as far in advance as possible because they must prepare multiples of equipment, supplies, forms, and so forth.
9. Preparation for full-scale resuscitation is completed at the start of the delivery.
10. Nursing personnel are alerted to the probability of an immediate postpartum hemorrhage.
11. Whether the woman requires an episiotomy depends on the estimated fetal weights, the anticipated need for manipulation if there are fetal malpresentations, and the relaxation of the perineum. An episiotomy may be cut at any time during the delivery.
12. Presentation and position of the babies is known before the start of delivery.
13. First twin is delivered in accord with its presentation and position.
14. An assistant directs the second twin into position abdominally as you deliver the first twin.
15. Quickly and securely clamp and cut the cord. There must be no delay in this action because the second twin may exsanguinate by bleeding through the cord if the twins are monozygotic.
16. Determine the presentation and position of the second twin and evaluate the size of this baby.
17. Closely monitor the fetal heart and scrutinize the vagina for any sign of bleeding while waiting for labor to resume. As long as there is no bleeding or evidence of fetal distress, haste is not indicated. The optimum time for the second twin to be born is between 3 and 15 min after delivery of the first twin, which allows the baby to come through the just fully dilated cervix before it starts to close again. Also, the second twin should be delivered before the placenta starts to separate.
18. Whether or not labor resumes within the time limit, the presenting part is guided into the true

pelvis by a combination of abdominal pressure and vaginal manipulations. Care is first taken to rule out a presenting umbilical cord.

19. Once the presenting part is fixed into the pelvis, rupture the membranes. If the presenting part is a breech or an unengaged head, leave your hand in the vagina to ascertain whether the cord has prolapsed. There is less chance of a prolapsed cord if the membranes are ruptured with no pressure (contractions or fundal) behind them and if they are leaked rather than torn.

20. Encourage the mother to push.

21. If the contractions still have not resumed and the maternal pushing effort is insufficient, an IV of 1000 mL D_5W or D_5RL with 10 IU of oxytocin added should be hung and started at a slow drip (1–2 mU/min).

22. Delivery is conducted as usual.

23. Third-stage hemorrhage or immediate postpartum hemorrhage is likely.

Uterine Inversion[18]

Predisposing Factors

Uterine atony

Patulous, dilated cervix

Fundal pressure or cord traction after the baby is born

Management

Call for physician backup

Establish patent IV

Treat for shock

Transfer into hospital if not there

Reposition uterus

If unable to reduce inversion, wrap exposed uterus in warm saline packs

Type and crossmatch

Repositioning the uterus is done with the placenta still attached. Blood loss is usually related to the length of time the uterus is inverted but is less if the placenta is removed *after* the uterus is replaced. Manual repositioning is accomplished by placing one entire hand in the vagina with the fingertips around the circumference of the junction where the uterus has turned on itself and the inverted fundus in the palm of the hand. Pressure is then applied with the palm of the hand on the fundus and the fingertips on the uterine walls. The fingertips walk up the uterine walls as the fundus is repositioned. Care must be taken not to puncture or rupture the soft uterine wall. At the same time the entire uterus is lifted high out of the pelvis, above the level of the umbilicus, and held there for several minutes. This puts tension on the uterine ligaments, which keeps the uterus reinverted.

Third-Stage Hemorrhage[19]

- Secondary to partial separation of the placenta from the uterine wall
- Most common reason is massage of the uterus before placental separation
- Identified by steady vaginal bleeding with the placenta still in the uterus, and determined to not be fully separated

Management

1. Have given a STAT call to your consulting physician.
2. If out of hospital, prepare for ambulance transfer.
3. Thoroughly massage uterus while applying controlled cord traction.
4. Simultaneously direct nurse or assistant to:
   - Establish patent IV
   - Hang Ringer's lactate or other appropriate crystalloid

- Draw type and crossmatch
- Monitor for shock

5. Manually remove the placenta (catheterize bladder first).
6. If unable to remove manually, add oxytocin to the IV.

Immediate Postpartum Hemorrhage (pph)[20]

Predisposing Factors

- Overdistended uterus
- Induction or augmentation of labor with oxytocin
- Rapid or precipitous labor and delivery
- Prolonged labor
- Grand multiparity
- History of uterine atony or pph

Management

- Evaluate consistency of uterus and massage
- Bimanual compression
- Simultaneously order oxytocics
- Assure patent IV; add oxytocic
- Consider other medications (Methergine, Prostin, or Hemabate)
- If no resolution, STAT call to consulting physician
- Verify type and crossmatch drawn or have it drawn
- Monitor blood pressure and pulse for shock
- Check placenta for completeness
- Explore uterus for missing placental fragments
- Examine for lacerations
- If shock ensues, place woman in shock position, cover warmly, administer oxygen, obtain and administer whole blood

TABLE 12-2   *Oxytocics: Standard Single Doses*

Drug	Dose	Route
Pitocin*	10 IU/mL	IM
Oxytocin*	10 IU/mL	IM
Syntocinon*	10 IU/mL	IM
Methergine‖	0.2 mg/mL	IM
	0.2 mg tab	PO
Prostin/15 M§	0.25 mg/mL	IM
Hemabate§	250 µg/mL	IM

*May be added to IV fluids. *Should never be given IV push.*

‖*Never give prior to birth of baby. Do not give IV.*

§Deep IM only.

Notes

Chapter 13

Postpartum[1]

Early Postpartum Examination

Chart Review

- Record of AP and IP course
- Number of hr/days postpartum
- Previous orders and progress notes
- Record of postpartal temperature, pulse, respirations, and blood pressure
- Laboratory and adjunctive study reports
- Medications record
- Nurses' notes

History

- Ambulation
- Voiding
- Bowel movements
- Appetite
- Discomforts/pain
- Concerns
- Questions
- Infant feeding

- Response to baby
- Reaction to labor and delivery

Physical Examination
- Blood pressure, temperature, pulse
- Throat, if indicated
- Breasts and nipples
- Auscultation of lungs, if indicated
- Abdomen: bladder, uterus, diastasis
- CVA tenderness
- Lochia: color, amount, odor
- Perineum: edema, inflammation, hematomas, pus, wound separation or dehiscence, stitches coming out, bruising; hemorrhoids
- Extremities: varicosities, calf tenderness and heat, edema, Homan's sign, reflexes

Management of Early Puerperium Care
- Ambulation/bed rest
- Diet
- Perineal care
- Voiding/catheterization
- Pain medication, prn
- Sleep medication, prn
- Laxative, prn
- Methergine 0.2 mg po q 4 hr × 6 doses then tid × 3 days, if indicated
- Discontinue IV, if applicable
- Supplementary vitamins or iron, or both, if indicated
- Relief measures for postpartum discomforts
- Breast care measures
- Laboratory screening for complications, if indicated
- Contraception plan
- Rh immune globulin, if indicated
- Rubella vaccine 0.5 mL SQ, if indicated

Fundal Height and Uterine Involution

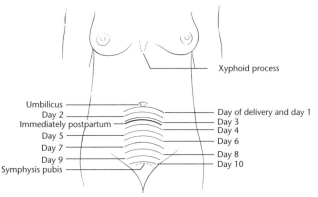

FIGURE 13-1   Fundal Height and Uterine Involution.[2]

Notes

Postpartum Complications
Puerperal Morbidity
Definition: Temperature $\geq$ 100.4°F occuring on any 2 of the first 10 days postpartum, excluding the first 24 hrs, taken by mouth at least four times daily.

Differential diagnosis
- Dehydration
- UTI
- Upper respiratory infection (URI)
- Mastitis

Puerperal Infection
Predisposing causes
The following circumstances predispose a woman to puerperal infection:

- Prolonged labor, especially with ruptured membranes
- Prolonged rupture of the membranes
- Numerous vaginal examinations during labor, especially with ruptured membranes
- Breaks in aseptic technique
- Carelessness regarding hand washing
- Any intrauterine manipulation (e.g., internal fetal monitoring, uterine exploration, manual removal of the placenta)
- Extensive tissue trauma, either as an open wound or as tissue devitalization
- Hematoma
- Hemorrhage, especially if more than 1000 mL of blood are lost
- Operative delivery
- Retention of placental fragments or membranes
- Improper perineal care
- Untreated vaginal/cervical infection or sexually transmitted disease (e.g., bacterial vaginosis, chlamydia, gonorrhea)

The classic clinical picture that predisposes a woman to puerperal infection is trauma accompanied by hemorrhage and maternal exhaustion.

General signs and symptoms

- Elevated temperature
- Tachycardia
- Pain

Infected Lower Genital Tract Trauma

Signs and symptoms

- Localized pain
- Dysuria
- Low-grade fever or sudden spike
- Edema
- Inflammation at wound site
- Pus, gray-green exudate
- Dehiscence
- Ulceration of old lesions

Treatment

- Remove any sutures
- Open, debride, and clean the wound
- Administer broad-spectrum antimicrobial drug
- Consult physician if necessary

Endometritis

Signs and symptoms

- Tachycardia, 100–140 bpm
- Temperature, 101°F to 104°F
- Chills
- Uterine tenderness extending laterally
- Increased afterbirth pains
- Subinvolution
- Abdominal distention
- Lochia scant and odorless, or heavy, foul, bloody, and seropurulent

- Onset 3 to 5 days postpartum, except with streptococcal infection
- Elevated WBC count

Treatment
- Hospital admission
- Physician consultation
- Broad-spectrum antimicrobial drug or triple antibiotic therapy, usually administered IV
- Discharge after being afebrile for 24 hours

Mastitis

Signs and symptoms

PRECURSORS
- Low-grade fever
- Mild pain in one breast quadrant, exacerbated when nursing
- Flu-like symptoms

MASTITIS
- Rapid temperature elevation to 103°F–104°F
- Increased pulse
- Chills, malaise, headache
- Breast area reddened, tender, painful, with hard lumps

BREAST ABSCESS
- Pus
- Remittent fever with chills
- Swollen, painful breast

Intervention
- Frequent breastfeeding and emptying of the breast
- Supportive bra
- Meticulous hand washing and breast care
- Warm compresses and massage
- Increased fluid intake
- Rest
- Stress and fatigue reduction

- Antibiotics
  - Dicloxacillin, or other penicillinase-resistant penicillin
  - Cephalosporins
  - Erythromycin, if allergic to penicillins

Thrombophlebitis

Signs and symptoms

SUPERFICIAL THROMBOPHLEBITIS

- Slight elevation of pulse and temperature
- Leg pain
- Localized heat
- Tenderness and redness

DEEP VENOUS THROMBOPHLEBITIS

- High fever, tachycardia, chills
- Abrupt onset of severe leg pain
- Edema of ankle, leg, thigh
- Positive Homan's sign
- Pain with calf pressure
- Tenderness along the affected vessel

Management

- Ultrasound venous study
- Bed rest
- Elevation of the extremity
- Heat
- Elastic stockings
- Analgesia
- Physician consultation for anticoagulant and/or antibiotic therapy

Pulmonary Embolus (Notify Physician STAT)

Signs and symptoms

- Sharp chest pain
- Shortness of breath, air hunger, tachypnea, dyspnea
- Respiratory rales

- Tachycardia
- Hemoptysis
- Apprehensiveness

Hematoma

Signs and symptoms

VAGINAL/VULVAR
- Perineal, vaginal, urethral, bladder, or rectal pressure
- Severe pain
- Tense, fluctuant swelling
- Blue to blue-black discoloration

BROAD LIGAMENT
- Lateral uterine pain, sensitive to palpation
- Flank pain
- Bulge felt on high rectal examination
- Ridge of tissue palpable laterally above the pelvic brim
- Abdominal distention

Subinvolution

Signs and symptoms
- Soft uterus with delayed or absent decrease in fundal height
- Persistent reddish brown lochia, or slow progress through the stages of lochial discharge followed by intermittent bleeding

Management
- Assess for infection
- Ergonovine (Ergotrate) 0.2 mg po q 4 hr × 3 days, or
- Methylergonovine (Methergine) 0.2 mg po q 4 hr × 3 days
- Reevaluate in 2 wk

Postpartum Depression

Symptoms

- Lack of ability to concentrate
- Loss of previous goals and interests; empty feeling
- Unbearable loneliness; feeling that no one understands
- Insecurity; need to be mothered herself
- Obsessive thinking about being a bad mother
- Lack of positive emotions
- Loss of self from fear that normalcy is irretrievable
- Loss of emotional control
- Anxiety attacks; feeling that she is on the edge of insanity
- Guilt and fear at thoughts of harming infant
- Thoughts of death

See also *Screening for Depression* on pp. 54–55.

Notes

Chapter 14

Newborn[1]

Immediate Care of the Newborn[2]
This refers specifically to care of the newborn in the initial minutes of life.

- Establish a clear airway
  - Hold baby's head lower than body with head turned to the side for drainage
  - Wipe the face and head, wiping fluid from the nose and mouth
  - Suction nasal and oral passages with a soft bulb syringe
- Keep the baby warm
  - Wipe and dry the baby
  - Place the baby on the mother's abdomen
  - Put a stockinet hat on the baby's head
  - Use a radiant warmer
  - Wrap the baby in warm blankets
- Show the infant to the parents and others, place on mother's abdomen if not already there
- Clamp and cut the umbilical cord
- Assign the 1 min and 5 min Apgar scores
- Immediate gross examination of the baby

TABLE 14-1   The Apgar Scoring System

	Score		
Sign	*0*	*1*	*2*
Heart rate	Absent	Slow, < 100	> 100
Respiratory effort	Absent	Slow, irregular	Good crying
Muscle tone	Flaccid	Some flexion of extremities	Active motion
Reflex irritability	None	Grimace	Vigorous cry
Color	Pale blue	Body pink, extremities blue	Completely pink

Source: Reprinted by permission from V. Apgar. The newborn (Apgar) scoring system: reflections and advice. *Ped Clin NA* 113:645 (August), 1966.

TABLE 14-2   Signs of Respiratory Compromise[3]

Visible Signs	**Audible Signs**
More than 60 rpm	Rales or rhonchi on auscultation
Cyanosis of face and trunk	
Nasal flaring	Stridor with inspiration
Retractions of intercostal muscles	Grunting on expiration
Retractions of sternum	
Apnea	

rpm = respirations per minute

TABLE 14-3   Signs of Normal Transition[4]

Assessment	Normal Value
Tone	Predominantly flexed
Sucking reflex	Intact
Behavior	Alertness alternating with sleep
Bowel sounds	Present after 30 min
Pulse	120–160 bpm; may vary with sleep or crying from 100 to 180 bpm
Respirations	30–60 rpm; diaphragmatic with abdominal wall movement
Temperature	Axillary: 36.5°C–37°C (97.7°F–98.6°F) Skin: 36°C–36.5°C (96.8°F–97.7°F)
Dextrostix	> 45 mg%
Hematocrit	< 65%–70%

Notes

Newborn Laboratory Values

Normal Newborn Heelstick Values
- Dextrostix, 45 mg% to 130 mg%
- Hematocrit, 45% to 65%

Cord Blood Values

TABLE 14-4   Cord Blood Values of a Full-Term Newborn

Component	Optimal Range
Hemoglobin concentration	14.0–20.0 g/dL
Red blood cell (RBC) count	4.2–5.8 million/mm^3
Hematocrit	43%–63%
Mean cell diameter	8.0–8.3 μm
Mean corpuscular volume (MCV)	100–120 μm^3
Mean corpuscular hemoglobin (MCH)	32–40 pg
Mean corpuscular hemoglobin concentration (MCHC)	30%–34%
Reticulocyte count	3%–7%
Nucleated red blood cell count	200–600/mm^3
White blood cell count	10,000–30,000/mm^3
Granulocytes	40%–80%
Lymphocytes	20%–40%
Monocytes	3%–10%
Platelet count	150,000–350,000/mm^3
Serum iron concentration	125–225 μg/dL
Total iron-binding capacity	150–350 μg/dL

Source: Reprinted by permission from A. Fanaroff and R. Martin. *Neonatal and Perinatal Medicine: Diseases of the Fetus and Infant,* 5th ed. St. Louis: Mosby, 1992, p. 943.

Normal Blood Gases

TABLE 14-5   Normal Blood Gases Immediately After Birth

Measurement	Normal Range
pH	
Umbilical artery	7.20–7.43
High altitude	7.20–7.42
Umbilical vein	7.26–7.48
pCO$_2$ (mm Hg)	
Umbilical artery	30–40
High altitude	23–65
Umbilical vein	25–50
pO$_2$ (mm Hg)	
Umbilical artery	4–37
High altitude	6.8–33
Umbilical vein	15–47
HCO$_3$ (mEq/L)	
Umbilical artery	15–27
High altitude	16.7–28
Umbilical vein	16–25
O$_2$ sat (%)	
Umbilical artery	2.2–71
High altitude	3.6–68.6
Umbilical vein	18.5–83.5

Data from Carlo and Waldemar, 1991; Dimich et al, 1991; Yancey et al, 1992; Yeomans et al, 1985.

Source: Reprinted by permission from S. Kelley (ed.), *Pediatric Emergency Nursing,* 2nd ed. Norwalk, CT: Appleton & Lange, 1994, p. 156.

Newborn Resuscitation

FIGURE 14-1   *Decision Making in Neonatal Resuscitation.*

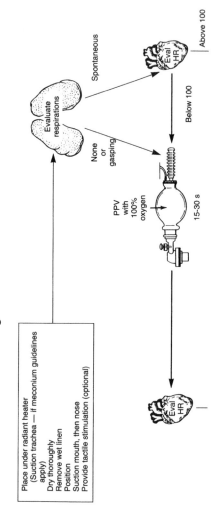

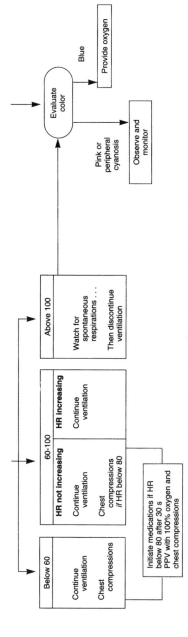

FIGURE 14-1 Decision Making in Neonatal Resuscitation. (continued)

Source: Reproduced with permission. © *Textbook of Neonatal Resuscitation*, 1987, 1990, 1994. Copyright American Heart Association.

PPV = positive pressure ventilation

HR = heart rate

s = seconds

Procedure for Positive Pressure Ventilation[5]

Equipment

1. Anesthesia bag with pressure gauge (manometer) *or* self-inflating bag with oxygen reservoir attachment
2. Infant- and premature-size face masks
3. Stethoscope
4. Feeding tube
5. Source of humidified oxygen with flow meter

Method

See *Precautions* that follow before beginning procedure.

1. Suction nares and oropharynx to clear secretions.
2. Place infant's head in a neutral position (when hyperextended, air enters esophagus).
3. Place mask over nose and mouth, making sure seal is tight.
4. Pressure for first breath should be 40–50 cm H_2O.
5. Subsequent breaths need about 25 cm H_2O or the lowest pressure that will allow you to see the chest wall expanding.
6. Ventilate 40–50 times per min for 2–3 min.
7. Have assistant auscultate anterior upper lobes of the lungs for aeration.
8. Continue to provide free-flow O_2 by face mask after infant has established respirations.

Precautions

1. Inadequate ventilation may be caused by poor seal around mask, flexed or hyperextended neck, or inadequate pressure of ventilation.
2. Face mask pressure near the infant's eyes can cause tissue damage.
3. Positive pressure ventilation will cause air retention in the stomach. After bagging for a brief period of time, vent the stomach by passing a feed-

ing tube. Any gastric contents should also be emptied. If bagging is going to continue over time (e.g., while awaiting a transport team), stop momentarily to slip a tube into the stomach to vent the stomach and prevent or reduce distention. Secure tube in place while continuing to ventilate.

Endotracheal Intubation[6]

Equipment
1. DeLee suction catheters
2. Endotracheal tubes, various sizes with adapters
3. Laryngoscope with blades
4. Positive pressure bag
5. Towel
6. Tape

Method

See *Precautions* that follow before beginning procedure.

1. Place infant with head in slightly extended position; may place towel under infant's shoulders.
2. Introduce laryngoscope at the right corner of the mouth.
3. Advance laryngoscope 2 to 3 cm while rotating it to midline and moving tongue to left.
4. When tip of blade is between the base of the tongue and the epiglottis, a slight elevation of the blade will expose the glottis (sometimes a gentle compression of the external larynx by an assistant will more easily expose the glottis).
5. Insert the endotracheal tube at the right side of the mouth and through the vocal cords, being sure you can easily see the tube (the tube must be small enough to allow an air leak, i.e., room around it; this space ensures easy expiration and reduces the risk of tissue damage).
6. Suction secretions if needed.

7. When the endotracheal tube is inserted, hold it firmly but gently in place and withdraw the laryngoscope slowly.
8. Attach the endotracheal tube to the adapter on the bag.
9. Ventilate with oxygen by bag; assistant should check for adequate ventilation of both lungs with stethoscope.

Precautions

1. If you have difficulty with the procedure, remove laryngoscope and ventilate with mask; try again in 2 min.
2. If tube is passed too far into the airway, it enters into the mainstem bronchus and breathing sounds on the left decrease. If this occurs, withdraw the tube slowly until breath sounds on the left increase.
3. If tube is left in place, suction as necessary with a sterile suction catheter when excess secretions are detected (possibly every 30–60 min).

Notes

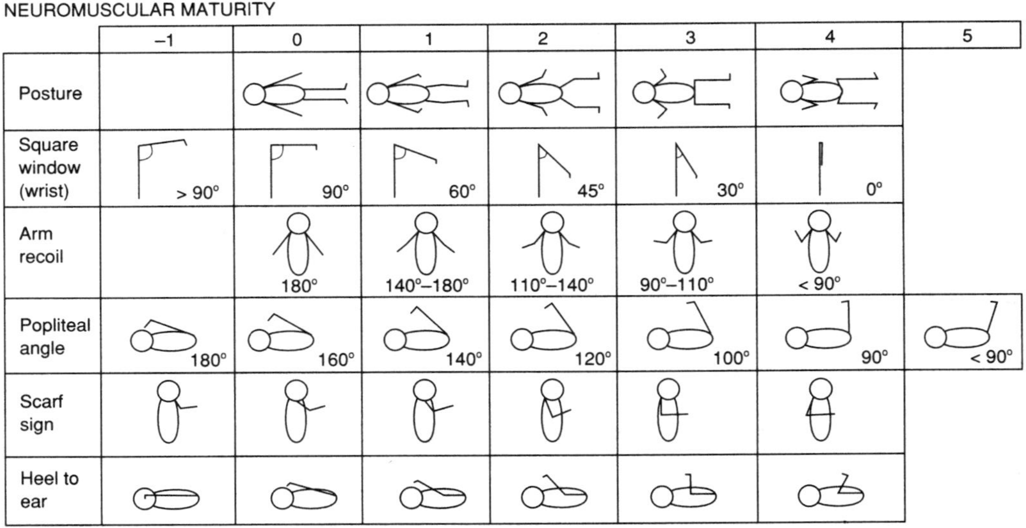

Gestational Age Assessment

NEUROMUSCULAR MATURITY

	−1	0	1	2	3	4	5
Posture							
Square window (wrist)	> 90°	90°	60°	45°	30°	0°	
Arm recoil		180°	140°–180°	110°–140°	90°–110°	< 90°	
Popliteal angle	180°	160°	140°	120°	100°	90°	< 90°
Scarf sign							
Heel to ear							

FIGURE 14-2 The New Ballard Scale (NBS).

continued.

PHYSICAL MATURITY

	−1	0	1	2
Skin	Sticky, friable, transparent	Gelatinous, red, translucent	Smooth, pink, visible veins	Superficial peeling and/or rash, few veins
Lanugo	None	Sparse	Abundant	Thinning
Plantar surface	Heel-toe 40–50 mm: −1 < 40 mm: −2	> 50 mm, no crease	Faint red marks	Anterior tranverse crease only
Breast	Imperceptible	Barely perceptible	Flat areola, no bud	Stippled areola, 1–2 mm bud
Eye/Ear	Lids fused loosely: −1 tightly: −2	Lids open; pinna flat, stays folded	Slightly curved pinna, soft, slow recoil	Well-curved pinna, soft but ready recoil
Genitals (male)	Scrotum flat, smooth	Scrotum empty, faint rugae	Testes in upper canal, rare rugae	Testes descending, few rugae
Genitals (female)	Clitoris prominent, labia flat	Clitoris prominent, labia minora small	Clitoris prominent, labia minora enlarged	Labia majora and minora equally prominent

FIGURE 14-2   The New Ballard Scale (NBS)
(continued)

3	4	5
Cracking, pale areas, rare veins	Parchment, deep cracking, no vessels	Leathery, cracked, wrinkled
Bald areas	Mostly bald	
Creases anterior two-thirds	Creases over entire sole	
Raised areola, 3–4 mm bud	Full areola, 5–10 mm bud	
Pinna formed and firm, instant recoil	Thick cartilage, ear stiff	
Testes down, good rugae	Testes pendulous, deep rugae	
Labia majora large, labia minora small	Labia majora cover clitoris and labia minora	

MATURITY RATING

Score	Weeks
−10	20
−5	22
0	24
5	26
10	28
15	30
20	32
25	34
30	36
35	38
40	40
45	42
50	44

FIGURE 14-2 The New Ballard Scale (NBS) (continued)

Source: Reproduced with permission from J. Ballard. New Ballard Scale, expanded to include extremely premature infants. *J Pediat* 119:417, 1991.

Clinical Manifestations of Hypoglycemia in the Newborn

- Episodes of tremors
- Cyanosis
- Seizures
- Apnea
- Limpness
- Irregular respirations
- Listlessness
- Difficulty in feeding
- Exaggerated Moro reflex
- Irritability
- High-pitched cry
- Coma

Types of Jaundice[7]

Physiological

- Jaundice not visible in first 24 hr
- Bilirubin rises slowly and peaks at day 3 to 4 of life
- Total bilirubin peaks at < 13 mg/dL
- Lab tests reveal predominance of unconjugated bilirubin
- Not visible after 10 days

Possible Pathological

- Jaundice visible during first 24 hr
- Bilirubin may rise quickly: > 5 mg/dL/24 hr
- Total bilirubin > 13 mg/dL
- Greater amounts of conjugated bilirubin
- Visible jaundice persists after 1 wk

Factors in Feeding History Requiring Immediate Evaluation[8]

- Regular projectile vomiting
- Bile-stained vomit
- No stools since birth
- No urination since birth
- Poor muscle tone—"spread-eagle posture"

- Inability to rouse infant
- Inability of infant to suck
- Rapid respirations over time (> 60 per min)
- Marked color changes during eating
- Taut, swollen abdomen
- More than six stools in 24 hr
- Bloody or excessively watery stools

TABLE 14-6 Nonspecific Signs of Illness in the Newborn[9]

Abnormal Physical Sign	Possible Etiology
Tachycardia (heart rate > 170 bpm)	Overheating
	Infection
	Anemia
	Shock
	Cardiac defect
Tachypnea (respirations > 60 rpm after transition)	Overheating
	Pulmonary disease
	Metabolic acidosis
	Cardiac disease
	Congenital defects of ribs, airway, lungs
Pallor	Cold stress
	Shock
	Anemia
Jaundice	Infection (prenatal or postnatal)
	Hemolytic disease
	Congenital defects of liver, biliary tract
	Abdominal obstruction
Abnormal cry	Central nervous system abnormalities
	Congenital defects of upper airway
Jitteriness	Hypoglycemia
	Hypocalcemia
	Drug withdrawal
	Normal variation
Feeding difficulties	Neuromuscular problems
	Infection
	Cardiac disease
	Respiratory disease
	Drug withdrawal

Your New Baby—the First Few Days

Eating

Your baby will probably be hungry every 2 to 4 hours around the clock. To help your baby adjust to a schedule like yours, wake him or her to feed every 3 to 4 hours when you are awake. Babies need only breast milk or formula for the first six months. Feeding your baby anything else will not help him or her to sleep better and may cause an allergic reaction. Remember to help the baby burp up swallowed air after each feeding (whether formula or breast milk).

Sleeping

Babies need a lot of sleep. To help your baby sleep when you want to sleep, provide a restful atmosphere and minimize interruptions or stimulation. Place your baby on his or her side or stomach to sleep.

Bowel Movements

Babies have greenish-black sticky stool for the first two days or so. This is called meconium. Breastfed babies' stool will then become golden-green, soft, and seedy-looking. Bottle-fed babies have dark brown, pasty, or formed stools. Your baby may have one to four stools a day. If your baby goes without a bowel movement for more than 2 days, contact your pediatrician or nurse-practitioner.

Voiding

Your baby should wet at least 4 to 5 diapers per day. This may be hard to tell if you are using paper diapers. If you have questions, use cloth.

FIGURE 14-3   *Example of Written Instructions To Be Sent Home with Family. (continued)*

Skin Care

Wash your baby with mild soap such as Ivory or Dove. Do not immerse the baby completely until the cord stump has fallen off and dried. This will happen in 1 to 2 weeks. Before then, wipe around the base of the cord with alcohol to help dry it out. Fold the front of the baby's diaper down so that the cord is not irritated by it. When changing diapers, wash the baby's bottom with soap and water. Avoid using powder and perfumed creams to help prevent diaper rash.

Safety

It is Pennsylvania and New Jersey State law that babies ride in car seats. Keep your baby as safe as he or she has been for the first nine months! Newborns can roll, so they must never be left unattended on changing tables, dressers, tables, or beds. Do not keep pillows, stuffed animals, quilts, and extra blankets in the baby's crib, because they can prevent the baby from getting enough air to breathe.

Danger Signs

Contact your pediatrician or nurse-practitioner immediately if:

- The baby becomes listless, will not eat, or behaves in an unusual way.
- The baby does not urinate within the first 24 hours.
- The baby has no bowel movement for 48 hours.
- The cord starts to smell bad or has pus oozing from it.
- The baby's temperature is below 97 degrees or above 99 degrees when taken under the baby's arm.
- The whites of the baby's eyes become yellow and the skin color looks yellow, tan, or peach.

FIGURE 14-3   *Example of Written Instructions To Be Sent Home with Family. (continued)*

Newborn Home Assessment

As your baby adjusts to life outside of your uterus, he or she will undergo many changes. To ensure that the changes your baby is experiencing are normal, it is helpful to check each of the following twice a day. Report any variations from normal to your midwife or physician.

	Day 1		Day 2		Day 3	
	9 AM	5 PM	9 AM	5 PM	9 AM	5 PM
Temperature Take under the baby's arm for 3–5 minutes. The temperature should be between 97° and 99°.						
Skin Check for jaundice or yellowing in the skin and whites of the eyes. Look at the baby in daylight near a window. Press on the baby's nose or breastbone; note the skin color when you release the pressure.						
Urination Note each time the baby has a wet diaper. There should be 5 or more a day.						
Bowel Movement Note color and number of bowel movements.						
Feeding The baby should be nursing or feeding every 2 to 3 hours for 15 to 20 minutes (2 to 4 ounces).						
Cord should become black and hard. Any pus or blood oozing from the stump is abnormal.						

FIGURE 14-3   Example of Written Instructions To Be Sent Home with Family. (continued)
Source: Used with permission of The Birthing Suite, Pennsylvania Hospital, Philadelphia, PA.

Notes

TABLE 14-7 *Recommended Schedule for Immunizations of Infants and Children*

Age	Vaccines	Comments
Newborn	HBV	First dose of HBV is administered before hospital discharge
2 mo	DTP	DTP may be given as early as 6 wk of age, then at 4- to 8-wk intervals for the first three doses
	OPV	
	HbCV	HbCV may be given as either HbOC or PRP-OMP
	HBV	Second dose of HBV may be given between 1 and 2 mo
4 mo	DTP	
	OPV	
	HbCV	HbCV may be given as either HbOC or PRP-OMP
6 mo	DTP	
	OPV	Optional dose of OPV, but recommended in high-risk areas
	HbCV	If HbOC was used, recommend another dose at 6 mo
	HBV	Third dose of HBV may be given between 6 and 18 mo
	HbCV booster	
12 mo		If PRP-OMP was used previously, recommend a HbCV booster dose given at 12 mo as the third dose of PRP-OMP

Age	Vaccine	
15 mo	MMR	MMR is usually not given to infants younger than 15 mo of age but may be given at 12 mo in high-risk areas
	HbCV booster	If HbOC was used previously, recommend another HbCV booster at 15 mo, which may be given as PRP-OMP, PRP-D, or HbOC
18 mo	DTP	DTP may be given between 15 and 18 mo, but usually between 6 and 12 mo after the third dose, and may be given simultaneously with MMR at 15 mo
	OPV	OPV may be given simultaneously with MMR and HbCV at 15 mo or any time between 12 and 24 mo
4–6 yr	DTP	DTP, OPV, and MMR at or before entry to kindergarten or elementary school; DTP can be given up to seventh birthday
	OPV MMR	AAP recommends the administration of the second dose of MMR at 11–12 years of age
14–16 yr	Td	Repeat every 10 years throughout life

HBV, Hepatitis B virus vaccine; DTP, diphtheria toxoid, tetanus toxoid, whole-cell pertussis vaccine; OPV, oral poliovirus vaccine; HbCV, Hemophilus b conjugate vaccine (three preparations are available: PRP-D [ProHIBiT], polyribosylribitol phosphate conjugated to diphtheria toxoid; HbOC [HibTITER], polyribosylribitol phosphate oligosaccharide conjugated with a nontoxic mutant diphtheria toxin; PRP-OMP [PedvaxHIB], polyribosylribitol phosphate conjugated with an outer membrane protein of N. meningitidis); MMR, measles, mumps, rubella vaccine; Td, tetanus toxoid (full dose) and adult strength diphtheria toxoid.

Source: Reprinted with permission of C. Poon. Childhood Immunization: Part 1. J. Pediatr. Health Care 6(6): 370, 1992.

Notes

References

All references listed below are from Helen Varney, *Varney's Midwifery,* 3rd ed. Boston: Jones and Bartlett Publishers, 1997. All material has been reprinted or adapted with permission.

Chapter 1
1. P. 25–28.

Chapter 2
1. P. 792.
2. P. 793.
3. P. 850.
4. P. 401.
5. Pp. 406–407; 440–441.

Chapter 3
1. Pp. 30–32.
2. Pp. 32–38.
3. Pp. 719–729.
4. Pp. 753–780.
5. Pp. 753–780.
6. P. 68.
7. Pp. 101–112.
8. Pp. 113–126.
9. P. 118.
10. Pp. 127–131.
11. Pp. 124–125.
12. M. E. Rousseau, pp. 214–215.
13. M. E. Rousseau, p. 215.
14. Pp. 215–216.

Chapter 4
1. N. Reedy, pp. 176–177.
2. Table 3.1, p. 46.
3. Pp. 45–46.
4. Pp. 48–49.
5. Pp. 49–51.
6. Pp. 51–60.
7. C. Krutsky et al, pp. 181–197.

Chapter 5
1. With N. Lachapelle, pp. 133–135.

Chapter 6
1. Pp. 253–257.
2. Pp. 257–258.
3. Pp. 231–232.
4. Pp. 250–251.
5. Pp. 255–256.
6. Pp. 259–260.
7. Pp. 257–258; 731–743.
8. P. 732.
9. P. 741.

Chapter 7
1. C. Gegor and J. Kriebs, pp. 283–316.
2. See pp. 292–293 for FMC charts.
3. Table 19.6, p. 296.
4. Table 19.7, p. 296.
5. Table 19.8, p. 296.
6. Table 19.10, p. 299.
7. Table 19.11, p. 299.
8. P. 304.

Chapter 8
1. Pp. 317–326.
2. Table 20.7, p. 325.

Chapter 9
1. A. Cowlin, pp. 149–165.

Chapter 10
1. With N. Reedy, pp. 327–377.
2. Pp. 327–329.
3. P. 331.
4. Pp. 331–333.
5. Pp. 334–337.
6. Pp. 337–340.
7. P. 340.
8. Pp. 341–343.
9. Table 21.1, p. 342.
10. Pp. 343–345.
11. Pp. 345–349.
12. Table 21.4, Pp. 347–348.
13. Pp. 349–350.
14. Pp. 350–352.
15. Pp. 352–356.
16. Table 21.7, p. 354.
17. Table 21.8, p. 355.
18. Pp. 359–364.
19. Table 21.9, p. 362.
20. Pp. 364–367.
21. P. 357.
22. Pp. 367–370.
23. Pp. 370–372.
24. Pp. 357–358.
25. P. 358.
26. Pp. 373–374.

Chapter 11
1. Pp. 381–524.
2. Pp. 381–383.
3. Pp. 397–400.
4. Table 23.1, p. 399.
5. Pp. 435–440.
6. Figure 24.4, p. 436.
7. Pp. 400–401.
8. Figure 23.7, p. 401.
9. Pp. 408–421.
10. Pp. 441–456.

11. P. 411.
12. Pp. 402–405.
13. Tables 23.4 and 23.5, p. 413
14. Pp. 421–431; 448–450.
15. P. 513
16. Pp. 835–840.

Chapter 12
1. Chapters 25 and 26.
2. Pp. 472–475.
3. Pp. 459–461.
4. Pp. 461–466.
5. L. Bertucci, pp. 476–483.
6. Figure 24.8, p. 440.
7. Figure 25.3, p. 482.
8. Pp. 483–485.
9. P. 485.
10. Pp. 485–487.
11. Pp. 487–488
12. P. 488.
13. Pp. 488–489.
14. Pp. 471–472.
15. Pp. 493–500.
16. Table 26.1, pp. 503–509.
17. Pp. 510–511.
18. Pp. 522–524.
19. Pp. 521–522.
20. Pp. 531–534.

Chapter 13
1. Pp. 623–683.
2. Figure 38.1, p. 624.

Chapter 14
1. M. K. McHugh, pp. 549–620.
2. Pp. 455–456.
3. Table 37.2, p. 610.
4. Table 33.3, p. 563.
5. Table 34.4, p. 575.
6. Table 34.5, p. 577.

7. Table 36.4, p. 607.
8. Table 36.3, p. 607.
9. Table 37.1, p. 610.

Appendix A
Sample Format for Chart Notes and Prescriptions

Revisit Antepartum Order of Report/Note*

Data Base:

_____ is a ___ year old Gravida ___ Para ___ currently at ___ weeks gestation by ___. She has been followed at _____ clinic since _____. At her initial visit: Family, Past Medical, Menstrual, and Reproductive Hx; PE, Pelvic, and Labs were significant for _____. Risks/Problems identified, pertinent f/u plans, and subsequent antepartal course _____.

Interval History Since Last Visit:

Client's subjective complaints or concerns
Headaches, visual disturbances, dizziness
Fever/chills, nausea/vomiting
Fetal movement, abdominal pain/contractions
Back pain, dysuria
Vaginal discharge, leaking fluid, bleeding
Constipation/hemorrhoids
Varicosities/leg ache, leg cramps
Edema (facial, hands, pretibial, ankle)
Exposure to any infectious diseases
Any relationship changes
Outcomes of labs, sonos, NSTs, consults, ER visits

Physical Findings Today:

Weight Gain ____ BP ____ Urine ____ CVAT ____
Fundal height and interval growth _____ EFW _____

Fetal Heart Rate/Rhythm/Location _____ Fetal Movement _____

Lie, Presentation, Position _____ Engagement ____

Edema _____ Reflexes _____

PRN Speculum: discharge, cultures, check for ROM

    Vaginal: effacement, dilatation, station, status of membranes

Assessment:

Size/Dates Concordance

Identified Problems and Risks

Plan: (Include as appropriate)

Diagnostic

Therapeutic

Educative

Consultation/Referral

RTC

*Sources: Mary Barger, CNM and *Varney's Midwifery, 3rd*, pp. 259–262.

Notes

Labor Admission Note

This is the ___(#)___ admission to ___(institution)___ of ___(name of patient)___, a ___(#)___ year old, gravida ____, para ____with an LMP of ____ and an EDB of ____ by _____ currently at ___(#)___ weeks gestation. No drug allergies. ABO/Rh: ___ CC: contractions which began at ___(time)___ and became regular at ___(time)___ at every ___(frequency)___. BOW _____. No history of vaginal bleeding. Last felt fetal movement at ___(time)___. With ___(significant others)___; coping _____.

Current Pregnancy History:

Past Obstetric History/Past Medical/Surgical/ GYN History/Family History/Social History:

(review from chart or do)

Physical Exam:

(review chart for full exam or do). Evaluate:

Vital signs: temperature/pulse/respirations
Uterine contractions: frequency/duration/intensity
Fetal heart: baseline rate/periodic changes/variability
Estimated fetal weight:
Fundal height:
Fetal position:

Pelvic Exam:

(in absence of PROM)

Cervix: position/effacement/dilatation
Station:
Presenting part:
Clinical pelvimetry:

Assessment:

Plan:

Delivery Note

  NSVD (or other type of delivery)   of a live   (#)   gram   (sex)   with Apgars ____ from   (position)   over (intact perineum/degree laceration/type episiotomy)   under (type anesthesia) . Placenta and membranes delivered spontaneously complete and intact.   (#)   cord vessels. Episiotomy/laceration repaired with (# and type of suture) . EBL of   (#)   cc. Oxytocin 10 IU IM (or whatever for uterine contraction).

Prescription Format

Name and dosage of medication, type and amount, route, number of times per day, number of days to be taken

Number of pills to be dispensed

Example:

  Amoxicillin 500 mg
  tab i po tid × 10 days
  #30

Notes

Postpartum Note (1–3 days)*

Hours/days pp _____ Breast _____ Bottle _____

Hx: ambulation
    voiding/bowel movements
    appetite
    rest/sleep
    discomforts/concerns
    questions about labor and delivery experience
    relationship/interaction with baby
    comfort with baby feeding and care
PE: Vital signs (TPR) _____ BP _____
    throat, if indicated
    heart: auscultation, if indicated
    lungs: auscultation, if indicated
    breasts: consistency (soft; filling; engorgement/hard)
                temperature
                nipple soreness; cracks
                presence of colostrum/milk
    abdomen: uterus: location, fundal height, size,
                        consistency, tenderness
                bladder: distention, retention, tenderness
                diastasis recti: when muscles tight and when
                        muscles relaxed
                bowel: distention, bowel sounds, when
                        indicated
    back: CVA tenderness
    extremities: varices, calf tenderness and heat, Homan's
                sign, edema, reflexes (if indicated)
    lochia: color, amount, clots, odor
    perineum: edema, inflammation, hematoma, pus,
                wound separation or dehiscence, stitches
                coming out, bruising
    hemorrhoids: number, size, internal/external, pain
Lab: (as indicated after initial note)
    Hct _____ ABO/Rh _____ PPD _____ VDRL _____
    Rubella _____ Varicella _____ HbsAg _____
    Chlamydia _____ Gonorrhea _____ Other _____

Diagnosis:

Plan:
*Varney's Midwifery, 3rd, pp. 635–637.

Notes

Appendix B
ACNM Documents

Contact the ACNM (see p. 352) for a list of other essential ACNM documents.

Definition of a Certified Nurse-Midwife

A certified nurse-midwife (CNM) is an individual educated in the two disciplines of nursing and midwifery, who possesses evidence of certification according to the requirements of the American College of Nurse-Midwives.

Accepted January 1978

Definition of Nurse-Midwifery Practice

Nurse-Midwifery practice is the independent management of women's health care, focusing particularly on pregnancy, childbirth, the postpartum period, care of the newborn, and the family planning and gynecological needs of women. The Certified Nurse-Midwife practices within a health care system that provides for consultation, collaborative management or referral as indicated by the health status of the client. Certified Nurse-Midwives practice in accord with the *Standards for the Practice of Nurse-Midwifery,* as defined by the American College of Nurse-Midwives.

Revised and approved by ACNM Board of Directors, July 27, 1992.
Revised August 22, 1993.

Philosophy of the American College of Nurse-Midwives

Nurse-midwives believe that every individual has the right to safe, satisfying health care with respect for human dignity and cultural variations. We further support each person's right to self-determination, to complete information and to active participation in all aspects of care. We believe the normal processes of pregnancy and birth can be enhanced through education, health care and supportive intervention.

Nurse-midwifery care is focused on the needs of the individual and family for physical care, emotional and social support and active involvement of significant others according to cultural values and personal preferences. The practice of nurse-midwifery encourages continuity of care; emphasizes safe, competent clinical management; advocates non-intervention in normal processes; and promotes health education for women throughout the childbearing cycle. This practice may extend to include gynecological care of well women throughout the life cycle. Such comprehensive health care is most effectively and efficiently provided by nurse-midwives in collaboration with other members of an interdependent health care team.

The American College of Nurse-Midwives (ACNM) assumes a leadership role in the development and promotion of high quality health care for women and infants both nationally and internationally. The profession of nurse-midwifery is committed to ensuring certified nurse-midwives are provided with sound educational preparation, to expanding knowledge through research and to evaluating and revising care through quality assurance. The profession further ensures that its members adhere to the Standards of Practice for Nurse-Midwifery in accordance with the ACNM philosophy.

Revised and approved October, 1989.

Standards for the Practice of Nurse-Midwifery

Nurse-midwifery practice is the independent management of women's health care, focusing particularly on pregnancy, childbirth, the postpartum period, care of the newborn, and the family planning and gynecological needs of women. The Certified Nurse-Midwife (CNM) practices within a health care system that provides for consultation, collaborative management or referral as indicated by the health status of the client. Certified nurse-midwives practice in accord with the Standards for the Practice of Nurse-Midwifery, as defined by the American College of Nurse-Midwives (ACNM).

The nurse-midwife is committed to maintaining a high standard of professional care, to participating in the education of nurse-midwives, and to promoting the concepts of nurse-midwifery practice in the community.

Standard I

*Nurse-midwifery care is provided
by qualified practitioners*

The practitioner:
1. Is certified by the ACNM approved certifying agent.
2. Shows evidence of continuing competency as required by the American College of Nurse-Midwives.
3. Is in compliance with the legal requirements of the jurisdiction where the nurse-midwifery practice occurs.

Standard II

*Nurse-midwifery care supports individual rights and
self-determination within boundaries of safety*

The certified nurse-midwife:
1. Practices in accord with the **Philosophy** and the **Code of Ethics of the American College of Nurse-Midwives.**
2. Provides clients with a description of the scope of nurse-midwifery services and information regarding the client's rights and responsibilities.
3. Provides clients with information on other providers and services when requested or when care required is not within the scope of the individual nurse-midwife.

4. Promotes involvement of support persons in the practice setting.

Standard III

Nurse-midwifery care is comprised of knowledge, skills, and judgments that foster the delivery of safe and satisfying care

The certified nurse-midwife:

1. Collects and assesses client care data, develops and implements a plan of management, and evaluates the outcome of care.
2. Demonstrates the clinical skills and judgments described in the ACNM **Core Competencies for Basic Nurse-Midwifery Practice.**
3. Practices in accord with the ACNM **Standards for the Practice of Nurse-Midwifery.**
4. Practices in accord with the policies of the nurse-midwifery service/practice that meet the requirements of the particular institution or practice setting.
5. Expands clinical practice in accordance with **ACNM Guidelines for the Incorporation of New Procedures into Nurse-Midwifery Practice.**

Standard IV

Nurse-midwifery care is based upon knowledge, skills, and judgments which are reflected in written policies/practice guidelines

The certified nurse-midwife:

1. Describes the parameters for the service/practice for nurse-midwifery management, physician management and collaborative management.
2. Establishes practice guidelines for each specialty area, which include but are not limited to:

Antepartum
   a) criteria for admission to the nurse-midwife service.
   b) parameters and methods for assessing the progress of pregnancy.

c) parameters and methods for assessing fetal well-being.
d) indicators of risk in pregnancy and appropriate intervention.
e) parameters for medications prescribed/used during pregnancy.

Intrapartum

a) parameters and methods for assessing progress of labor and birth.
b) parameters and methods for assessing maternal and fetal status.
c) parameters for medications and solutions prescribed/used during labor and birth.
d) management of birth and the immediate postpartum period.
e) methods to facilitate the newborn's adaptation to extrauterine life.
f) significant deviations from normal and appropriate interventions.
g) parameters and methods for assessing the immediate well-being of the newborn.

Postpartum/Newborn

a) parameters and methods for assessing the postpartum status of the mother.
b) parameters and methods for assessing the well-being of the newborn.
c) parameters for medications prescribed/used in the puerperium.
d) significant deviations from normal and appropriate interventions.

Family Planning/Gynecology

a) parameters and methods for assessing general physical and emotional status of the client.
b) parameters for medications and devices prescribed/used.
c) significant deviations from normal and appropriate interventions.

Standard V

Nurse-midwifery care is provided in a safe environment

The certified nurse-midwife:

1. Demonstrates knowledge of and utilizes federal and state regulations that apply to practice environment and infection control.
2. Promotes adequate staffing in the clinical setting where the nurse-midwife practices.
3. Demonstrates appropriate techniques for emergency management including arrangements for emergency transportation.

Standard VI

Nurse-midwifery care occurs within the health care system of the community using appropriate resources for referrals to meet medical, psychosocial, economic, and cultural or family needs

The certified nurse-midwife:

1. Demonstrates a safe mechanism for obtaining medical consultation, collaboration and referral.
2. Uses community services.
3. Demonstrates knowledge of medical, psychosocial, economic, cultural, and family factors that may affect care.

Standard VII

Nurse-midwifery care is documented in legible, complete health records

The certified nurse-midwife:

1. Uses records that facilitate communication of information to consultants and institutions.
2. Facilitates clients' access to their records.
3. Provides written documentation of risk assessment, course of management, and outcome of care.
4. Provides for prompt entry on the health record of laboratory tests, treatments, and consultations.

5. Provides a mechanism for sending a copy of the health record on referral or transfer to other levels of care.
6. Treats records as confidential documents.

Standard VIII

Nurse-midwifery care is evaluated according to an established program for quality assessment that includes a plan to identify and resolve problems

The certified nurse-midwife:

1. Participates in a program of quality assurance/improvement for the evaluation of nurse-midwifery practice within the setting in which it occurs and within legal requirements.
2. Collects client care data systematically and is involved in analysis of that data for the evaluation of the process and outcome of care.
3. Seeks consultation to review problems identified by the quality assurance/improvement program.
4. Acts to resolve problems that are identified.
5. Participates in peer review.

Notes

Guidelines for the Incorporation of New Procedures into Nurse-Midwifery Practice

Nurse-Midwifery practice will continue to evolve, depending on the needs of the client, the needs of the site, the expectations of the institution, and the nurse-midwife's desire to improve care to women and their families. Procedures incorporated into the practice of nurse-midwifery should be in concert with the **Philosophy of the American College of Nurse-Midwives** and the **Standards for the Practice of Nurse-Midwifery** of the American College of Nurse-Midwives (ACNM) and should not conflict with any current clinical practice statements of the ACNM.

While the ACNM does not approve or disapprove the incorporation of new clinical procedures into nurse-midwifery practice, the following guidelines were developed by the Clinical Practice Committee and approved by the Board of Directors to assist the nurse-midwife in expanding clinical practice:

1. Identify need for the procedure, taking into consideration:
   a) consumer demand
   b) safety considerations
   c) institutional request
   d) availability of qualified personnel
   e) interest of nurse-midwives
2. Cite relevant statutes/documents that would constrain or support incorporation of the procedure, including:
   a) statutes and regulations
   b) institutional bylaws
   c) legal opinions
3. Evaluate procedure as a nurse-midwifery function, including:
   a) relevant literature
   b) use by other nurse-midwives
   c) risks/benefits
   d) management of complications
4. Develop process for educating nurse-midwives to perform this procedure, using:

    a) bibliography
    b) formal study
    c) supervised practice
    d) protocols
    e) evaluation of learning

5. Evaluate use of procedure, documenting:
    a) outcome statistics
    b) satisfaction with procedure
      — consumer
      — institution
      — nurse-midwifery practice
    c) maintenance of competency

6. Any new procedure incorporated into nurse-midwifery practice will be done according to the "Guidelines for the Incorporation of New Procedures into Nurse-Midwifery Practice" as outlined in the *Standards for the Practice of Nurse-Midwifery* and reported on the form provided by the American College of Nurse-Midwives. The completed form shall be mailed to the ACNM for reporting purposes. Supporting documents, as outlined in the "Guideline," should be placed with the written policies of the nurse-midwifery practice/service (Standard IV).

Standards for the Practice of Nurse-Midwifery, Approved BOD August 1993; supersedes Functions, Standards, and Qualifications, 1983 and **Standards for the Practice of Nurse-Midwifery,** 1987. **Guidelines for the incorporation of New Procedures into Nurse-Midwifery Practice,** 1987; supersedes **Guidelines for Evaluation of Nurse-Midwifery Procedural Functions,** 1979 (Amended 10/90, 11/92)

©4/87 American College of Nurse-Midwives

Reporting Form for Guidelines for the Incorporation of New Procedures into Nurse-Midwifery Practice

The following information is solicited by the American College of Nurse-Midwives according to the directions contained in the Standards for the Practice of Nurse-Midwifery (1993) and the Guidelines for the Incorporation of New Procedures into Nurse-Midwifery Practice (1992). The purpose of this reporting form is to provide statistical information on the new procedures that nurse-midwives are incorporating into their practices.

Date _____

Name of CNM completing this form _____

Name of Nurse-midwifery service _____

Address _____

City/State/Zip _____

Phone(s) _____

Name and brief description of procedure _____

_____

_____

Number of CNMs at your site who have completed training to perform this procedure _____

❏ By checking this box, I give permission to ACNM to give my name to another certified nurse-midwife who may wish to contact my service about incorporating this procedure.

Please mail this form to:
Director of Professional Services and Support
American College of Nurse-Midwives
818 Connecticut Ave. NW Suite 900
Washington, DC 20006

REMINDER: Supporting documents as outlined in the Guidelines should be placed with the written policies of the nurse-midwifery practice/service.

Approved by ACNM Board of Directors, February 1993

Appendix C
Street and E-mail Addresses, Telephone, Fax, and Beeper Numbers

American College of Nurse-Midwives (ACNM)
818 Connecticut Avenue, NW, Suite 900
Washington, D.C. 20006
Phone: 202-728-9860   FAX: 202-728-9897

Centers for Disease Control and Prevention (CDC)
1600 Clifton Road, NE
Atlanta, GA 30333
Phone: 404-639-3311   Internet: Http://www.cdc.gov

Appendix D
Computer Prompts and Passwords

Appendix E
Certificate and License Numbers

_____

_____

_____

_____

_____

_____

_____

_____

_____

_____

_____

_____

_____

_____

_____

_____

_____

_____

_____

Appendix F
Abbreviations and Acronyms

ABO	blood groupings based on the presence of antigens on the red cell surface
AC	abdominal circumference
AFI	amniotic fluid index
AFP	alpha-fetoprotein
AFV	amniotic fluid volume
AGA	average for gestational age
AIDS	acquired immunodeficiency syndrome
ALT	alanine aminotransferase
AP	antepartum
AST	aspartase aminotransferase
A-V	atrioventricular
BhCG	β human chorionic gonadotropin
bid	twice daily
BMI	body mass index
BMR	basal metabolism rate
BP	blood pressure
BPD	biparietal diameter
bpm	beats per minute
BPP	biophysical profile
BST	breast stimulation test
BSU	Bartholin's, skenes, urethra
BUN	blood urea nitrogen
BV	bacterial vaginosis
°C	degrees Centigrade
c/s	cesarean section
CBC	complete blood count
cc	cubic centimeter
CC	chief complaint

CDC	Centers for Disease Control and Prevention
CIN	cervical intraepithelial neoplasia
cm	centimeter
CMV	cytomegalovirus
CPD	cephalopelvic disproportion
CRL	crown-rump length
CST	contraction stress test
ctx	contractions
CVA	costovertebral angle; cerebrovascular accident
CVAT	costovertebral angle tenderness
D&C	dilatation and curettage
DES	diethylstilbestrol
dL	deciliter
DPT	diphtheria, pertussis, tetanus [vaccine]
DTR	deep tendon reflex
DUB	dysfunctional uterine bleeding
EAB	elective abortion
EBL	estimated blood loss
EDD (EDB, EDC)	estimated date of delivery (birth, confinement)
EFM	electronic fetal monitoring
EFW	estimated fetal weight
ELISA	enzyme-linked immunosorbent assay
°F	degrees Fahrenheit
FH	fundal height; fetal heart
FHR	fetal heart rate
FHT	fetal heart tones
FL	femur length
FMC	fetal movement counting
FSH	follicle-stimulating hormone
FTA/ABS	fluorescent treponemal antibody absorbed
f/u	follow up
g or gm	gram
GA	gestational age
GC	gonorrhea
G/P	gravida/para

G6PD	glucose-6-phosphate dehydrogenase
GTT	glucose tolerance test
h&h	hemoglobin and hematocrit
HbCV	hemophilus b conjugate vaccine
HBIG	hepatitis B immune globulin
HBV	hepatitis B virus
HC	head circumference
hCG	human chorionic gonadotropin
hct	hematocrit
HDL	high density lipoprotein
HELLP	hemolysis, elevated liver enzymes, low platelets
Hg	mercury
Hgb	hemoglobin
HGSIL	high grade squamous intraepithelial lesion
HIV	human immunodeficiency virus
HPV	human papillomavirus
HR	heart rate
HRT	hormone replacement therapy
hs	bedtime
HSV	herpes simplex virus
Hx	history
IgG	immunoglobulin G
IgM	immunoglobulin M
IM	intramuscular
IP	intrapartum
ISG	immune serum globulin
IU	international unit
IUD	intrauterine device
IUGR	intrauterine growth restriction
IUPC	intrauterine pressure catheter
IV	intravenous
kcal	kilocalorie, Calorie
kg	kilogram
KOH	potassium hydroxide
L	liter
LAA	left acromion anterior
LAP	left acromion posterior

lb	pound
LDH	lactate dehydrogenase
LDL	low density lipoprotein
LFT	liver function test
LGA	large for gestational age
LGSIL	low-grade squamous intraepithelial lesion
LH	luteinizing hormone
LMA	left mentum anterior
LMP	last menstrual period; left mentum posterior
LMT	left mentum transverse
LOA	left occiput anterior
LOP	left occiput posterior
LOT	left occiput transverse
LSA	left sacrum anterior
LSP	left sacrum posterior
LST	left sacrum transverse
MA	mentum anterior
MAP	mean arterial pressure
mcg (µg)	microgram
µU	microunit
MCH	mean corpuscular hemoglobin
MCHC	mean corpuscular hemoglobin concentration
MCV	mean corpuscular volume
mEq	milliequivalent
milliIU	milli international units
mg	milligram
ml	milliliter
mm	millimeter
mmol	millimole
MMR	measles, mumps, rubella vaccine
MMWR	Morbidity and Mortality Weekly Report
mOsm	milliosmol
MSAFP	maternal serum alphafetoprotein
MVP	mitral valve prolapse
MVU	Montevideo Units

ng	nanogram
NST	non-stress test
OA	occiput anterior
OC	oral contraceptive
OCT	oxytocin challenge test
OP	occiput posterior
OPV	oral polio vaccine
OT	occiput transverse
OTC	over-the-counter
O_2 sat	oxygen saturation
Pap	Papanicolaou
pCO_2	partial pressure of carbon dioxide
PCP	pneumocystis carinii pneumonia; primary care provider
PCR	polymerase chain reaction
PE	physical examination
pg	prostaglandin gel
PGE_2	prostaglandin E_2
$PGF_{2\alpha}$	prostaglandin F_{2alpha}
pH	measure of acidity or alkalinity
PID	pelvic inflammatory disease
PIH	pregnancy-induced hypertension
PMI	point of maximal impulse
PMP	prior menstrual period
PMR	perinatal mortality rate
PMS	premenstrual syndrome
pO_2	oxygen tension, partial pressure of oxygen
po	by mouth
PP	postpartum
PPD	purified protein derivative
PPH	postpartum hemorrhage
PPROM	preterm, premature rupture of membranes
PPV	positive pressure ventilation
prn	as needed
PROM	premature rupture of membranes
PT	prothrombin time
PTT	partial thromboplastin time

pv	in the vagina
qid	four times daily
qd	daily
qod	every other day
RAA	right acromion anterior
RAP	right acromion posterior
RBC	red blood cell [count]
RDA	Recommended Daily Allowance
Rh	Rhesus factor
RMA	right mentum anterior
RMP	right mentum posterior
RMT	right mentum transverse
ROA	right occiput anterior
ROM	rupture of membranes; range of motion
ROP	right occiput posterior
ROS	review of systems
ROT	right occiput transverse
rpm	respirations per minute
RPR	rapid plasma reagin
RSA	right sacrum anterior
RSP	right sacrum posterior
RST	right sacrum transverse
RTC	return to clinic
Rx	prescribe
s	seconds
SAB	spontaneous abortion
SGA	small for gestational age
SGOT	serum glutamic oxalacetic transaminase
SGPT	serum glutamic pyruvic transaminase
SIL	squamous intraepithelial lesion
SQ	subcutaneous
STD	sexually transmitted disease
Sx	symptom
TAB	therapeutic abortion
TB	tuberculosis
Td	tetanus-diphtheria vaccine
TIBC	total iron binding capacity

tid	three times daily
TPR	temperature, pulse, respirations
TSH	thyroid-stimulating hormone
UA	urinalysis
UPI	uteroplacental insufficiency
URI	upper respiratory infection
UTI	urinary tract infection
VBAC	vaginal birth after cesarean
VDRL	Venereal Disease Research Laboratory
VIN	vulvar intraepithelial neoplasia
VZIG	varicella zoster immune globulin
WBC	white blood cell [count]
ZDV	Zidovudine

Notes

Appendix G
FDA Pregnancy Risk Categories for Drugs

A   Controlled studies in women fail to demonstrate a risk to the fetus in the first trimester (and there is no evidence of a risk in later trimesters), and the possibility of fetal harm appears remote.

B   Either animal reproduction studies have not demonstrated a fetal risk but there are no controlled studies in pregnant women, or animal reproduction studies have shown an adverse effect (other than a decrease in fertility) that was not confirmed in controlled studies in women in the first trimester (and there is not evidence of a risk in later trimesters).

C   Either studies in animals have revealed adverse effects on the fetus (teratogenic or embryocidal or other) and there are no controlled studies in women or animal studies are not available. Drugs should be given only if the potential benefit justifies the potential risk to the fetus.

D   There is positive evidence of human fetal risk, but the benefits from use in pregnant women may be acceptable despite the risk (e.g., if the drug is needed in a life threatening situation or for a serious disease for which safer drugs cannot be used or are ineffective).

X   Studies in animals or human beings have demonstrated fetal abnormalities or there is evidence of fetal risk based on human experience or both, and the risk of the use of the drug in pregnant women clearly outweighs any possible benefit. The drug is contraindicated in women who are or may become pregnant.

Source: Federal Register 44:37434–37467, 1980.

Appendix H

Temperature Conversion Chart

Centigrade*	Fahrenheit*
35.5	96.0
35.6	96.1
35.7	96.3
35.8	96.4
35.9	96.6
36.0	96.8
36.1	97.0
36.2	97.2
36.3	97.3
36.4	97.5
36.5	97.7
36.6	97.9
36.7	98.1
36.8	98.2
36.9	98.4
37.0	98.6
37.1	98.8
37.2	99.0
37.3	99.1
37.4	99.3
37.5	99.5
37.6	99.7
37.7	99.9
37.8	100.0
37.9	100.2
38.0	100.4
38.1	100.6

Centigrade*	Fahrenheit*
38.2	100.8
38.3	100.9
38.4	101.1
38.5	101.3
38.6	101.5
38.7	101.7
38.8	101.8
38.9	102.0
39.0	102.2
39.1	102.4
39.2	102.6
39.3	102.7
39.4	102.9
39.5	103.1
39.6	103.3
39.7	103.5
39.8	103.6
39.9	103.8
40.0	104.0

*rounded to the nearest 0.1 degree

Index

Abbreviations and acronyms, 356–61

Abdominal obstetric examination, 101–4

Abdominal rub in labor, 231

ABO and Rh disease, 196–97
nonroutine uses of antepartum Rh immune globulin, 197

Abortion, spontaneous
inevitable, 150–51
missed, 151–52
threatened, 149–50

Abruptio placentae, 194–95
management of hemorrhage in, 196

ACNM. *See* American College of Nurse-Midwives

AIDS. *See* HIV infection and AIDS

Alcohol abuse, screening for, 53–54

Alpha-fetoprotein (AFP) triple screen, 100

Amenorrhea, 60

American College of Nurse-Midwives (ACNM)
definition of certified nurse-midwife, 342
definition of nurse-midwifery practice, 342

guidelines for incorporation of new procedures into nurse-midwifery practice, 349–51
philosophy, 343
standards for the practice of nurse-midwifery, 344–48

Amnionitis, 250

Amniotic fluid index (AFI), 120–21, 121*t*

Amniotic fluid volume (AFV), 120–21, 121*t*

Amniotomy in cervical ripening, 237–38

Anaphylactic shock, 76–77

Anemia, 168–69, 172
laboratory findings in 169*t*, 170–71*t*

Antepartal complications, 149–204

Antepartum
charting, 336–37
clinical pelvimetry, 104
fetal heart tone location for specific fetal positions, 105
fundal heights during pregnancy, 102, 102*t*
initial history, 89–90
initial physical and pelvic examination, 92–93

laboratory tests and adjunctive studies, 100–101
Leopold's maneuvers, *103*
obstetric abdominal examination, 101
order of report, 336–37
pregnancy tests, 93–97, *94*, 97*t*
present pregnancy history, 90–92
revisits, 98–100
  chart review in, 98
  interval history in, 98–99
  laboratory tests and adjunctive studies in, 100–101
  physical examination in, 99–100
Apgar scoring system, 310*t*
Asthma, 175–76
Asynclitism, *219*, 219–20

Back rub in labor, 231
Bacterial vaginosis, 63–64
Ballard score, new, 319–21
Battledore placenta, 234
Biophysical profile, 113
  criteria for, 117*t*
  indications for, 116*t*
  modified, 120
  obstetrical management based on modified, 118–19*t*
Bishop's Score, 236–37, 236*t*
Bleeding. *See also* Hemorrhage
  dysfunctional uterine, 59–60
Blood transfusion reactions, 274–75
Bloody show, 212
Body mass index, 125, 126*t*, 127*t*
Bradycardia, fetal, 251–52

Breast, anatomy of, *9*
Breast cancer, monitoring for, 38
Breast examination
  charting of findings, 16–17
  findings, 14–16
  physical examination, 14
  relevant history, 14
  variations in
    postpartal woman, 17–18
    pregnant woman, 17
Breastfeeding
  and mastitis, 305–6
  nipples in, 18
Breathing exercises in labor, 229
Breech presentation, delivery of infant in a, 283–93

Calcium, dietary sources of, 135*t*
Caloric intake, determining, 125
Caloric requirements, calculating, during pregnancy, 132*t*
Candidiasis, 62–63
Cephalopelvic disproportion, 267–68
Certified Nurse-Midwife, definition, 342
Cervical infections, 62–64
Cervical ripening and induction of labor, 235–37
  Bishop's score, 236–37, 236*t*
  methods of, 237–38
Chadwick's sign, 94, 95
Chart notes, sample format for, 336–39
Chickenpox. *See* Varicella
Chlamydia, 65–66
Chorioamnionitis, 250
Chronic hypertension, 190
Clinical pelvimetry, 104

Cold compresses in labor, 231
Colostrum, 17
Combined Pawlik's grip, *104*
Condoms, use of, for HIV-
    positive women, 80–81
Condylomata acuminata (geni-
    tal warts), 73–75
Contraception
    effectiveness of methods in,
        26–27*t*
    emergency postcoital contra-
        ception, 40–43
    intrauterine contraceptive
        devices (IUDs), 27–30
    long-term hormonal contra-
        ception
        Depo-Provera, 37–39
        Norplant (levonor-
            gestrel), 39–40
    oral hormonal contraception,
        30–36
Contractions
    assessment of, 226, 228
    hypertonic uterine, 270–71
    hypotonic uterine, 270
Contraction stress test, 114–15
Conversion chart, 364
    Fahrenheit to Centigrade, 364
    Pounds and ounces to grams,
        inside back cover
Coombs' test-antibody titer, for
    Rh negative women,
    196–97
Cord compression, causes of,
    258
Cystocele, 19

Deep transverse arrest, 268–69
Delivery
    in breech presentation,
        283–93
    and eclampsia, 191

in face presentation, 281–83
    management of, 223–24
Delivery note, 339
Depo-Provera, 37–39
Depression
    postpartum, 308
    screening for, 54–55
Diabetes mellitus, 176–77, 180
    diagnoses based on labora-
        tory tests and indicated
        management, 179*t*
    management plan for screen-
        ing, 178*t*
Dietary guidelines for women
    with gestational diabetes,
    108–81
Diethylstilbesterol, screening of
    women with intrauterine
    exposure to, 58
Differential diagnosis, process
    of, 3
Down Syndrome
    and elevation of maternal
        serum alpha-fetopro-
        tein, 107
    risk of, by maternal age, 108*t*
Drug safety categories, 362
Dysfunctional uterine bleeding,
    59–60

Eclampsia, 183, 190
    delivery considerations, 191
    emergency management of
        seizures, 190–91
Ectopic pregnancy, 153–54
Edema, 184
    gestational, 183
Effleurage in labor, 231
Emergency postcoital contra-
    ception, 40–43
Endocarditis, 174–75, 174*t*
Endometritis, 304–5

Endotracheal intubation, 317–18

Enterocele, 19

Estimated date of delivery, calculating, 96

Exercise during pregnancy
  management of, 142
  medical screening, *144*
  prenatal matenal activity chart, 145*t*–148*t*
  safety issues, 143

Exhaustion, prevention of, in labor, 229

Estrachorial placenta, 233–34

Face presentation, delivery of infant with a, 281–83

False labor, 207, 212

Family planning. *See* Contraception

Fanning in labor, 230

Fetal assessment
  amniotic fluid volume (AFV), 120–21, 121*t*
  biophysical profile (BPP), 117–120
    criteria for, 117*t*
    indications for, and suggested testing frequency, 116*t*
    modified, 120
    obstetrical management based on modified, 118–19*t*
  contraction stress test, 114–15
    indications for, 114
    interpretation criteria, 114–15
    management of results, 115
  fetal movement counting,

111, 111–12

genetic counseling, 108
  conditions calling for, 110*t*
  maternal serum alpha-fetoprotein (MSAFP) levels in, 107–08

nonstress test, 112–13
  indications for, 112
  interpretation criteria for, 113*t*
  management of results, 113

obstetrical ultrasound
  components of basic, 123
  indications for, 122
  indications for limited, 123–24

triple screen, 107

Fetal distress, 264–65

Fetal heart, auscultation in labor, 226

Fetal heart rate
  acceleration patterns, 254
  assessment of, 226
  bradycardia, 251–52
  deceleration patterns, 254–65
  early decelerations, 254–55
  late decelerations, 256–58
  minimal or absent variability, 252–53
  prolonged deceleration, 261–62
  sinusoidal pattern, 262–64
  tachycardia, 251
  variability minimal or absent, 252–53
    short-term, long-term, classification, 224–25
  variable decelerations, 258–61

Fetal heart tones, points of maximum intensity of, for specific fetal positions, *105*

Fetal monitoring in labor, 224, 225

Fetal movement counting, *111*, 111–12

Fetal skull, 8–9

Folic acid
    dietary sources of, 136–37*t*
    preconception use of, 87
    supplementation, 134

Follicle stimulating hormone (FSH), laboratory values, 4

Food guide pyramid, 139, *139*

Fundal height
    antepartum, *102*, 102*t*
    postpartum, *302*

Gastrointestinal changes, during first and second stages of labor, 11

Genetic counseling, 108, 110*t*

Genital warts, 73–75

Gestational edema, 183

Gestational hypertension, 183

Gestational proteinuria, 183

Glucose-g-phosphate dehydrogenase (G6PD) deficiency, 172

Glycosuria, 177

Gonorrhea, 66–68

Goodell's sign, 95

Gravida, determining, 89–90

Health history and examination
    breast examination in, 14–18
    laboratory tests and adjunctive studies

for the nonpregnant woman, 20, 22–25*t*
    for the pregnant woman, 22–25*t*
    pelvic examination, 18–20
    routine history, 13
    routine physical examination and review of systems, 13–14

Heart disease, 172–75

Hegar's sign, 95

HELLP syndrome, 187

Hematologic changes, during first and second stages of labor, 11

Hematoma, 307

Hemoglobin/hematocrit, 20

Hemoglobinopathies, 168–69

Hemorrhage. *See also* Bleeding
    immediate postpartum, 298
    third-stage, 297–98

Hepatitis, 156
    history, 156–57
    laboratory evaluation, 157
    physical examination, 157
    precautions to avoid exposure to, 160
    viral hepatitis A, 157–58
    viral hepatitis B, 158–59

Herpes simplex virus (HSV), 71–73

Higgins nutritional intervention methodology, 127, 128*t*, 129*t*, 130–32

History
    antepartal, 89–90
    and breast examination, 14
    in hepatitis, 156–57
    intrapartal, 205–8
    past medical history, 207
    in perimenopausal women, 45–46
    postpartum, 300–301

in pregnancy diagnosis, 94–95

present pregnancy, 90–92, 206

routine, 13

HIV infection and AIDS, 78–84

care of women with early HIV infection, 81–82

condom use, 80–81

counseling and testing, 78–79

in labor, 83

laboratory tests, 79

in the newborn, 84

in pregnancy, 82–83

routes of transmission, 78

safety of sexual activities, 79–81

Hormonal contraception. *See* Long-term hormonal contraception; Oral hormonal contraception

Hormone replacement therapy, 47–49

commonly prescribed regimens, 50–51*t*

Hydatidiform mole, 152–53

Hydramnios, 200–202

Hyperemesis gravidarum, 175

Hypertension, 183–84

chronic, 190

gestational, 183

Hypertensive disorders of pregnancy, 182–87

eclampsia, 183

gestational edema, 183

gestational hypertension, 183

gestational proteinuria, 183

preeclampsia, 182, 183–85

Hyperthyroidism, 182

Hypertonic uterine contractions, 270–71

Hypoglycemia, clinical manifestations in newborn, 322

Hypothyroidism, 181–82

Hypotonic uterine contractions, 270

Immunizations

recommended schedule for infants and children, 328–29*t*

for rubella, 162

for varicella, 163–64

Inevitable abortion, 150–51

Infection, puerperal, 303–4

Intrapartum. *See also* Delivery; Labor

complications in, 235–299

laboratory tests, 211

Intrauterine contraceptive devices (IUDs)

absolute contraindications, 28

in emergency postcoital contraception, 43

management of syncope, 29

pregnancy with, in place, 29–30

relative contraindications, 28

safety measures for insertion, 29

types of, 27

Intrauterine growth restriction (IUGR), 199–200

Intrauterine pressure, evaluation of, 226, 228

Intravenous infusion, indications for, 224

Iron

dietary sources of, 133*t*

supplementation, 133, 133*t*

IUDs. *See* Intrauterine contraceptive devices (IUDs)

Jaundice in newborn, 322–23

Ketoacidosis, 271–72

Labor
  admission note, 338
  and asynclitism, *219,* 219–20
  cervical ripening and inductions of, 235–38, 236*t*
  contractions, 226, 228
  diagnosis of, and initial evaluation, 205–11
    history, 205–8
    laboratory tests, 211
    pelvic examination, 210–11
    physical assessment, 208–10
  false, 212
  fetal heart rate, assessment, 224–26
  first stage of
    management plan for normal, 221–22
    physiological changes during, 10–11
  herpes simplex virus and, 72–73
  HIV infection and AIDS and, 83
  indications for intravenous infusion, 224
  length of, 212–13
  lie, presentation, position, and variety, 214, 215*t*
  management of delivery, 223–24

  mechanisms of, 216–22
  medications commonly given in, 227*t*
  physiological changes during, 10–11
  preterm, 241–48
  progress in, 212–13
  second stage of
    management plan for, 222–23
    physiological changes during, 10–11
  signs and symptoms of impending, 211–12
  support and comfort measures in, 228–33
  and synclitism, 219–20
  third stage of
    placenta and cord variations, 233–34
    signs of placental separation, 233
Large-for-gestational-age fetus, 177
Leg cramps, alleviation of, during labor, 232
Leopold's maneuvers, 101, *103,* 281
Lie, 214, 215*t*
Lightening, 211
Luteinizing hormone (LH), laboratory values, 4

Management framework
  principles, 2
  process, 1
  skills, 2–3
Mantoux test, 155–56
Mastitis, 305–6
Maternal exhaustion, 271–72
Maternal serum alpha-fetoprotein (MSAFP), 107–110

Mauriceau-Smellie-Veit maneuver, 291–293
Medical screening for prenatal exercise participants, *144*
Medications
  interactions with oral contraceptives, 34–35*t*
  in labor, 227*t*, 231
Menstrual cycle, 5
Missed abortion, 151–52
Mitral valve prolapse, antibiotic prophylaxis, 173*t*
Mole, hydatidiform, 152–53
Monilia, 62–63
Montevideo units (MVU), 228
Montgomery's follicles or tubercles, 17, 94–95
Morbidity, puerperal, 303
Mouth care in labor, 230
Multiple gestation, 293–96

Naegele's rule, 96
Neonatal herpes, 73
Neonatal resuscitation, decision making in, *314–15*
Neural tube defect, and use of folic acid, 87
Newborn
  Apgar scoring system for, 310*t*
  gestational age assessment, 319–21
  HIV infection and AIDS in, 84
  home assessment, *326*
  hypoglycemia in, 322
  immediate care of the, 309
  immunizations, recommended schedule, 328–29*t*
  instructions for family, *324–25*

jaundice in, 322–23
  laboratory values for, 312
  cord blood values of full-term, 312*t*
  normal blood gases immediately after birth, 313*t*
  nonspecific signs of illness in, 323*t*
  resuscitation, 314–18
    decision making, 314–15
    endotracheal intubation, 317–18
    positive pressure ventilation, 316–17
    signs of normal transition in, 311*t*
    signs of respiratory compromise in, 310*t*
Nipple stimulation in cervical ripening, 237
Nonstress test, 112–113, 113*t*
Norplant (levonorgestrel), 39–40
Nurse-midwife, certified, 342
Nurse-midwifery practice
  definition of, 342
  guidelines for incorporation of new procedures into, 349–51
  standards for, 344–48
Nutritional high-risk populations, identifying, 132
Nutrition
  dietary sources of
    calcium, 135*t*
    folic acid, 134, 136–37*t*
    iron, 133, 133*t*
    protein, 132*t*, 138*t*
    vitamin C, 134, 134*t*
  food guide pyramid, *139*

weight gain in pregnancy
  body mass index, 125, 126*t*,
    127*t*
  Higgins intervention method-
    ology, 127, 128*t*, 129*t*,
    130–32

Occiput anterior position,
    216–18
Occiput posterior position,
    218–19
Oligohydramnios, 202–3
Oral hormonal contraception
  absolute contraindications,
    30–31
  in emergency postcoital con-
    traception, 41, 43*t*
  interactions with selected
    medications, 34–35*t*
  noncontraceptive benefits, 30
  principles of pill switching, 36
  relative contraindications, 31
  side effects and complica-
    tions, 31, 32–33*t*
  warning symptoms of
    adverse reactions, 36
Osteoporosis prevention and
    therapy, 52
Oxytocics, 299*t*
Oxytocin, in cervical ripening,
    238
Oxytocin challenge test,
    114–15

Pap smear
  management of results,
    56–57*t*
  in screening women with
    intrauterine exposure
    to diethylstilbestrol, 58
Para, determining, 89–90
Pawlik's grip, *104*

Pelvic examination, 18
  defects of vaginal/rectal mus-
    culature, 19–20
  at onset of labor, 210–11
  types of speculae used in,
    18–19
Pelvic inflammatory disease
    (PID), 75–76
Pelvic inlet, diameters of, 6
Pelvimetry, clinical, 104
Pelvis
  bones of, 6
  planes and diameters, 7
  types of, 7
Perimenopausal women
  history, 45–46
  hormone replacement ther-
    apy for, 47–49
    commonly prescribed
      regimens, 50–51*t*
  laboratory tests and adjunc-
    tive studies, 46–47
  osteoporosis prevention and
    therapy, 52
  physical examination, 46
Perineal anatomy, *8*
Persistent posterior postion,
    218–19
Physical examination. *See also*
    Pelvic examination
  antepartal, 92–93
  in early postpartum examina-
    tion, 301
  at onset of labor, 208–10
  in perimenopausal woman,
    46
  in pregnancy diagnosis, 95
  routine, 13–14
Physiological changes during
    first and second stage
    labor, 10–11
Pill switching, principles of, 36
Pinard maneuver, 285–286

Piskacek's sign, 95, 96
Placenta
  battledore, 234
  extrachorial, 233–34
    circumvallata, 234
    marginata, 234
  previa, 193–94
    management of hemor-
      rhage in, 196
  separation, signs of, 233
  succenturiate, 233
Pneumonia, varicella, 163
Polyhydramnios, 177, 200–202
Positioning in labor, 229
Position of fetus, 214, 215*t*
Positive pressure ventilation in
    newborns, 316–17
Postdates pregnancy, 203–4
Postmaturity syndrome, 203–4
Postpartum
  breast examination in, 17–18
  complications, 303–8
  depression, 308
  early examination in,
    300–301
  fundal height and uterine
    involution, *302*
  management of early care,
    301
Postpartum note, 340
Preconception care, 86–87, 87*t*
Preeclampsia, 177, 182,
    183–90
  associated or predisposing
    conditions to, 184–85
  laboratory findings in,
    188–89*t*
  screening for, on each prena-
    tal visit, 185–86
  severe, 186–187, 190
  signs, classic, 183–184
Pregnancy. *See also* Antepar-
    tum; Prenatal

dating, 95–97, 97*t*
diagnosis of, 94–97
ectopic, 153–54
exercise during, 142–48,
    145*t*–48*t*
HIV infection and AIDS in,
    82–83
with IUD in place, 29–30
nutrition in. *See* Nutrition
tests, serum and urine, 93–94
weight gain in
  body mass index, 125,
    126*t*, 127*t*
  Higgins intervention
    methodology, 127,
    128*t*, 129*t*, 130–32
Premature rupture of the mem-
    branes, 212, 248–49
Prenatal maternal activity
    chart, 145*t*–148*t*
Prescription format, 339
Presentation, 214, 215*t*
Preterm labor, 241–48
  management of care,
    241–45
  signs and symptoms of,
    241
  tocolysis in, 245
Primary amenorrhea, 60
Privacy, assurance of, in labor,
    230
Protein
  dietary sources of, 138*t*
  requirements, during preg-
    nancy, 127–32
Proteinuria, 183–84
Puerperal infection, 303–4
Puerperal morbidity, 303
Pulmonary embolus, 306–7

Rectocele, 19
Relaxation exercises in labor,
    229

Respiratory compromise, signs of in newborn, 310*t*

Rest, provision of, in labor, 229

Rh negative women, in pregnancy, 196–97

Rubella, 161–62
antibody titer values, 161
malformations caused by, 161
management, 161
signs and symptoms, 161
vaccine, 162

Rupture of membranes (ROM), 211, 212, 237
premature, 248–49

Safety issues in exercise during pregnancy, 143

Secondary amenorrhea, 60

Seizures, emergency management of eclamptic, 190–91

Serum beta-hCG, in pregnancy tests, 93, *94*

Sexual intercourse in cervical ripening, 237

Sexually transmitted diseases, 64–65. *See also* HIV infection and AIDS
chlamydia, 65–66
condylomata acuminata (genital warts), 73–75
gonorrhea, 66–68
herpes simplex virus (HSV), 71–73
pelvic inflammatory disease (PID), 75–76
syphilis, 68–71
trichomonal vaginitis, 65

Shoulder dystocia, 278–81

Significant others during labor, 232

Size-dates discrepancy, 197–98

Skull, fetal, *8*
diameters of, *9*

Small for gestational age (SGA), 199–200

Speculae, types of, 18–19

Spontaneous abortion, 149–52

Subinvolution, 307

Synclitism, 219–20

Syncope, management of, 29

Syphilis, 68–71

T-ACE, 53

Tachycardia, fetal, 251

Third-stage hemorrhage, 297–98

Threatened abortion, 149–50

Thrombophlebitis, 306

Thyroid disease, 181–82

Tocolysis in premature labor, 245–46

Toxic shock syndrome, symptoms and prevention of, 58–59

Trichomonal vaginitis, 65

Triple screen in fetal assessment, 107–8
management of results, 109*t*

Trophoblastic disease, 184

Tubal pregnancy, 153–54

Tub bath in labor, 230

Tuberculosis, screening test, 155–56

Ultrasound
accuracy of pregnancy dating by, 97*t*
obstetrical, 122–24

Umbilical cord prolapse, 276–78

Urethrocele, 19

Urinary tract infections, 165

management of, 166–67*t*
Uterine contractions
 hypertonic, 270–71
 hypotonic, 270
Uterine descensus, 19–20
Uterine dysfunction, 269–71
Uterine inversion, 296–97
Uterine rupture, 272–73
 management, 273
 risk factors for, in vaginal
  birth after cesarean,
  240–41
 signs and symptoms of, 240,
  272–73
Uterine sizing, 96–97
Uteroplacental insufficiency
 causes of chronic and acute,
  256, 258
 causes of chronic fetal stress
  due to, 264
Uterus, positions of, *21*

Vaccines. *See* Immunization
Vaginal birth after cesarean
  (VBAC), 240–41
Vaginal examinations, support
  for, during labor, 231–32
Vaginal/rectal musculature,
  defects of, 19–20

Varicella, 162–65
 signs and symptoms, 163
 congenital syndrome, 162
 management of care of
  woman, 164–65
 maternal infection, 162–63
 signs and symptoms of pneumonia, 163
 transmission, 163
 vaccine for, 163–64
Variety, 214, 215*t*
Vasa previa, 234
Velamentous cord insertion,
  234
Viral hepatitis A, 157–58
Viral hepatitis B, 158–59
Vitamin C
 dietary sources of, 134*t*
 supplementation, 134
Vulvovaginal/cervical infections, 62–64

Warts, genital, 73–75
Weight gain during pregnancy,
  125–32

ZDV therapy, 82–84